THE
HERBAL REMEDIES
BIBLE

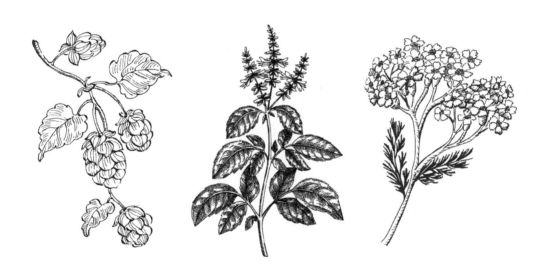

[7 IN 1]
THE COMPLETE GUIDE TO NATURAL MEDICINE

Unlock the Power of Herbs for Tinctures,
Essential Oils, Infusions, and Holistic Health Solutions.

AMBER WHITMORE

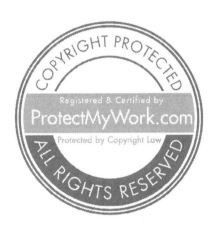

DISCLAIMER: The herbal remedies, recipes, and information contained in this book are provided for informational and educational purposes only. They are not intended to replace or substitute professional medical advice, diagnosis, or treatment. If you have or suspect you have a medical condition or are currently on medication, always consult with a qualified healthcare provider before starting any new treatment or regimen. The author and publisher of this book make no representation or warranties about the accuracy, reliability, completeness, or timeliness of the content. They assume no liability or responsibility for any errors or omissions in the content of this book, or for any adverse reactions, direct or indirect consequences resulting from the application of any of the advice, preparations, or procedures described herein.

Contents

INTRODUCTION

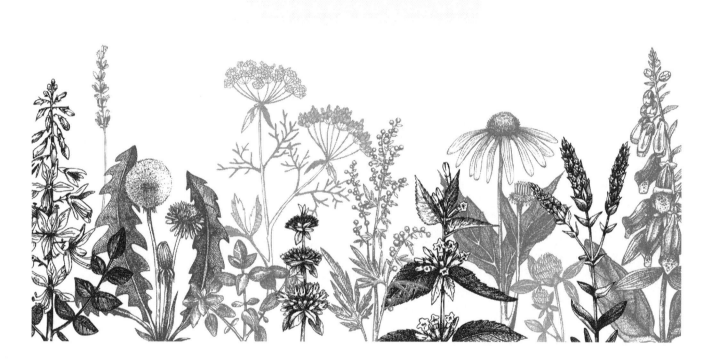

Herbal medicine has been an integral part of human history, shaping our understanding of health, wellness, and the natural world around us. From the ancient wisdom of traditional healers to the innovative practices of modern herbalists, using plants for healing has been a vital component of our collective journey toward better health. As we continue to navigate the complexities of modern life, herbal remedies offer an opportunity to reconnect with nature, balance our bodies, and cultivate a deeper understanding of our well-being.

I've always been fascinated by herbs and their healing power; by 'always,' I mean since I was a kid. In my childhood, I found myself immersed in a world where the secrets of herbs unfolded before my eager eyes. It was within the wise embrace of my grandmother that I discovered the timeless wisdom passed down through generations of our family. A formidable expert in herbs, she had acquired a profound understanding of their benefits, nurtured by her father's role as an herb importer. Through this privileged connection, she had the opportunity to explore and experience a vast array of herbs from all corners of the world. From the humblest leaves to the most exotic spices, she possessed a comprehensive knowledge of their healing potential. No illness, from a bothersome headache to the grip of a cold or even fearsome influenza, could withstand the power of her herbal concoctions.

As a child, I had the honor of being her apprentice, carefully cleaning and preparing the herbs, packaging them alongside her, and eagerly taking notes of her teachings while she told me everything about them in her aromatic kitchen. Those cherished moments have shaped who I am today. Now, as the author of this book, I stand ready to share with you the precious legacy of herbs entrusted to me.

One of my beautiful experiences as an herbalist occurred when my sister, Sarah, reached out for assistance with her unrelenting migraines. Doctors prescribed her various medications, but nothing seemed to relieve her. After a thorough consultation, I suggested that Sarah try a combination of feverfew and ginger, known for their efficacy in treating migraines. To our delight, the herbal remedy significantly reduced the frequency and intensity of her migraines, and she was able to regain control of her life.

After that incident, an overwhelming sense of pride and usefulness washed over me. I couldn't help but feel a deep sense of accomplishment and fulfillment, knowing I possessed a special knowledge about herbs that remained unknown to everyone else. This experience and countless others reaffirmed my belief in the boundless potential of herbal remedies to improve our quality of life.

This book contains a wealth of information gathered from centuries of herbal wisdom, as well as practical advice on how to make use of the healing power of plants. We will look at different herbs and their benefits in treating common ailments, managing chronic conditions, and boosting overall wellness. I will also share with you some of the most brilliant personal anecdotes and insights from my own experience as an herbalist to bring this fascinating world to life and make it more tangible for you.

As we start this adventure together, I hope you can appreciate nature's beauty and complexity even more. The plants around us aren't just pretty scenery - they're powerful gems that can help us stay healthy and happy. So let's get started to unveil the secrets of nature's healing power hidden within these pages!

BOOK I

EMBRACING NATURE'S WISDOM

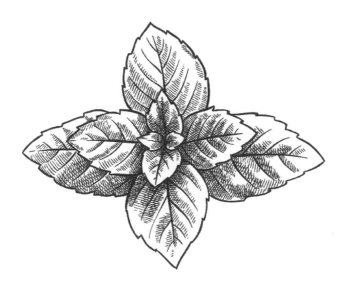

AMBER WHITMORE

Chapter One

The Evolution of Herbal Medicine

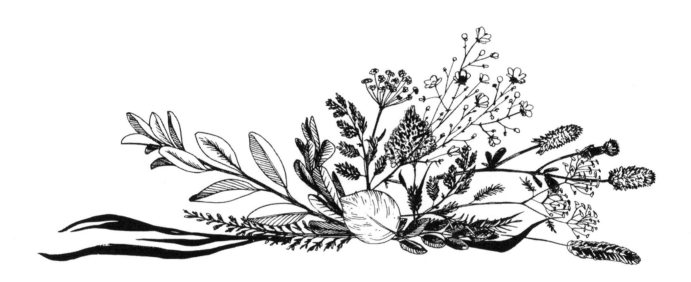

This book will take you on an exciting tour through the rich history of herbal medicine, the importance of herbal medicines in today's fast-paced world, and the critical components of safety and precautions that assure responsible use.

Learning about the history of herbal medicine allows us to better appreciate the valuable knowledge passed down by our ancestors. While herbal remedies are not a cure-all, it is crucial to recognize their potential healing benefits and practice responsible usage to ensure safety and effectiveness.

Origins of Herbal Medicine

Long before the advent of modern medicine, our ancestors relied on the healing properties of plants to address various ailments and maintain their well-being. The earliest evidence of plant-based remedies can be traced back thousands of years, providing insights into the origins of herbal medicine and the relationship between humans and the natural world.

Prehistoric Herbal Use

One of the earliest known examples of plant-based remedies comes from the remains of a Neanderthal burial site in modern-day Iraq, dating back approximately 60,000 years. This site's excavations showed the presence of eight plant species, many of which are still used for their therapeutic benefits today. Yarrow, chamomile, and marshmallow were among the herbs used for their anti-inflammatory, wound healing, and calming characteristics. This finding implies that our forefathers recognized the natural healing properties of plants and used them to improve their health.

Another fascinating example comes from the Ötzi the Iceman, a remarkably well-preserved mummy discovered in the Italian Alps dating back to around 3300 BCE. Analysis of Ötzi's belongings revealed the presence of a birch polypore mushroom, which has known antibacterial and antiparasitic properties. It is believed that Ötzi carried this mushroom to treat wounds or intestinal parasites, further underscoring the long-standing use of plants as natural remedies.

In addition to the direct application of plant-based remedies, shamanic and spiritual healing practices often incorporated the use of plants for both their physical and metaphysical properties. Ancient shamans and healers from various cultures around the world relied on the power of plants to facilitate spiritual journeys, cleanse negative energies, and restore balance within the body and mind.

A remarkable example involves using Ayahuasca by indigenous Amazonian cultures, a potent hallucinogenic concoction created from the Banisteriopsis caapi vine, and the leaves of the Psychotria Viridis plant. Ayahuasca has been used in shamanic rituals for thousands of years to facilitate profound spiritual experiences, promote psychological healing, and restore physical health.

Similarly, the indigenous peoples of North America have long used sage, cedar, and sweetgrass in spiritual ceremonies and smudging rituals. These plants are believed to have purifying and protective properties, helping to cleanse negative energy and promote spiritual well-being.

Ancient Civilizations

- Ancient Egyptian civilization profoundly understood the natural world and employed extensive herbal remedies for medical and spiritual purposes. The Ebers Papyrus, one of the oldest known medical texts dating back to 1500 BCE, contains over 700 plant-based remedies, highlighting the Egyptians' vast knowledge of herbal medicine. Some commonly used herbs in ancient Egypt included garlic, onion, coriander, and pomegranate, valued for their antibacterial, anti-inflammatory, and antioxidant properties.

- The ancient Greeks and Romans also contributed significantly to the development of herbal medicine. One of the most influential figures in this field was Hippocrates, often called the "Father of Medicine." Hippocrates is credited with systematizing medical knowledge, emphasizing the importance of observing patients and the natural course of diseases. He advocated using herbs such as willow bark, which contains salicin, a compound that led to the development of modern-day aspirin.

Another key figure in the Greek and Roman herbal tradition was Dioscorides, a Greek physician who served in the Roman army. His seminal work, "De Materia Medica," is a comprehensive compendium of over 600 plants and their medicinal uses, which would influence Western medicine for centuries to come.

- Ayurveda, a holistic system of medicine originating in ancient India over 5,000 years ago, emphasizes using herbs to maintain balance and harmony within the body. Rooted in the belief that good health comes from the equilibrium between the body, mind, and spirit, Ayurveda utilizes a diverse range of plants to address various health concerns. Some essential herbs in Ayurvedic medicine include Ashwagandha, known for its adaptogenic properties; turmeric, valued for its anti-inflammatory and antioxidant effects; and tulsi, or holy basil, revered for supporting respiratory health and alleviating stress.

- Traditional Chinese Medicine (TCM) is another ancient healing system that has extensively employed herbal remedies for thousands of years. TCM is based on the concept of Qi, or life force, which flows through the body along meridians, and the balance of Yin and Yang, representing opposing yet complementary strengths. To maintain harmony within the body, TCM practitioners prescribe various herbs tailored to the individual's unique constitution and the specific imbalance being addressed.

Some well-known herbs in TCM include ginseng, recognized for its adaptogenic and energy-boosting properties; astragalus used to support the immune system; and goji berries, famous for their antioxidant content and ability to improve vision.

Middle Ages and Renaissance

Herbal therapy advanced significantly during the Middle Ages and Renaissance periods. Monastic gardens, apothecaries, herbals, and early medical books arose as major elements of the changing landscape, while Islamic and Arabic medicine shaped the knowledge and practices of the time.

Monastic Gardens and Apothecaries

During the Middle Ages, monastic gardens were crucial for cultivating and studying medicinal plants. Monks, the primary keepers of knowledge during this period, maintained and expanded their gardens, providing a steady supply of herbs for the monastery and the surrounding community. Many monasteries had an adjoining apothecary, where medicinal herbs were processed, stored, and dispensed to needy people.

Herbals and Early Medical Texts

The Middle Ages and Renaissance also produced numerous "herbals," illustrated books describing plants and their medicinal properties. Herbals played a vital role in disseminating herbal knowledge, often drawing from the works of ancient Greek, Roman, and Islamic scholars. One of the most influential herbals of the period was the "Herbarum Vivae Eicones" by Otto Brunfels, a German botanist and theologian, which included detailed illustrations and descriptions of more than 300 plants.

Influence of Islamic and Arabic Medicine

The Islamic Golden Age, from the 8th to the 13th century, witnessed prominent advancements in various fields, including medicine. Islamic and Arabic scholars preserved and expanded upon the medical knowledge of the ancient Greeks and Romans, translating and commenting on key texts by Hippocrates, Galen, and Dioscorides. These scholars made major contributions to understanding herbal medicine by integrating knowledge from other cultures, such as Indian and Persian traditions.

The Persian polymath Al-Razi, sometimes known as Rhazes in the West, was a key figure in Islamic medicine. "Al-Hawi," his extensive medical encyclopedia, included a wealth of information on herbal medicines and notably influenced European medicine during the Middle Ages. Ibn Sina, often known as Avicenna, was a well-known Persian physician and philosopher. "The Canon of Medicine," his massive opus, had a detailed Materia Medica section describing over 800 medicinal compounds, many of which were derived from plants.

Herbal Medicine Today

The modern era has brought about dramatic changes in medicine, with the rise of modern pharmacology, the rediscovery of herbal medicine, and its integration with conventional healthcare. In this section, we will explore these developments and their impact on the practice of herbal medicine today.

The Rise of Modern Pharmacology

The advent of modern pharmacology in the 19th and 20th centuries revolutionized medicine with the development of synthetic drugs and the isolation of active compounds from natural sources. This period saw the discovery of numerous groundbreaking medications, many of which were derived from plants. For example, the isolation of morphine from the opium poppy (Papaver somniferum) in 1804 provided the foundation for developing a wide range of pain-relieving drugs. Similarly, the discovery of salicylic acid from willow bark led to the development of aspirin, one of the most widely used medications in the world.

Rediscovery of Herbal Medicine

Despite the rapid advancement of modern pharmacology, the latter half of the 20th century saw a resurgence of interest in herbal medicine, driven by growing concerns about the side effects of synthetic drugs and a desire to reconnect with nature. This period saw the establishment of organizations such as the American Herbalists Guild, dedicated to promoting the responsible use of herbal medicine and supporting the education of herbal practitioners.

The growing demand for natural remedies has resulted in the development of a diverse range of herbal products and supplements, making them readily accessible in health food stores and online markets.

Integration with Conventional Healthcare

As the popularity of herbal medicine has grown, efforts have been made to integrate herbal remedies with conventional healthcare practices. Many healthcare professionals now recognize the potential benefits of herbal medicine and incorporate it as a complementary therapy alongside conventional treatments. For example, ginger (Zingiber officinale) to alleviate nausea and vomiting associated with chemotherapy has become a widely accepted practice.

Furthermore, numerous research studies have been conducted to validate the efficacy and safety of herbal remedies, leading to a greater understanding of their potential benefits and risks. This scientific investigation has resulted in the development of standardized herbal extracts and the establishment of guidelines for the responsible use of herbal medicine.

The Future of Herbal Medicine

As we look toward the future of herbal medicine, it's essential to learn about the opportunities and challenges that lie ahead. By focusing on scientific research, sustainable practices, and the evolving role of herbalists, we can ensure that the traditions we cherish continue to grow and thrive in the modern world.

Scientific Research and Validation

The good news is that the growing scientific evidence supporting herbal treatment for numerous health issues is promising. This research helps doubters accept the field and enhances our understanding of how these natural medicines operate and how to utilize them responsibly and efficiently.

For example, ongoing studies on the benefits of turmeric (Curcuma longa) and its active compound, curcumin, have shed light on its anti-inflammatory properties. This research has led to a growing acceptance of turmeric as a valid option for managing chronic inflammation and pain, both in the general public and the medical community.

Sustainable Practices and Conservation

As the popularity and demand for herbal remedies grow, we must encourage the responsible use of these valuable plant resources. The increasing focus on permaculture and agroforestry practices involves cultivating medicinal plants to support the health of the surrounding ecosystems. By integrating herbal plants into diverse, sustainable agricultural systems, we can help protect the environment and, at the same time, meet the growing demand for natural remedies.

Ethical Foraging

Foraging, or the act of gathering these wild plants, is a timeless tradition that unites us with our ancestral roots, invites us to deepen our connection with the Earth, and opens doors to the rich world of herbal medicine. However, foraging requires not only knowledge and skill but also a deep sense of respect and responsibility for nature. This respect and responsibility manifest in the practice of ethical foraging.

Ethical foraging entails adopting practices prioritizing preserving nature and ensuring its continued bounty for future generations. It's like an unwritten pact between the Earth and us, a promise to maintain the delicate balance of ecosystems from which we draw our healing plants.

One fundamental principle of ethical foraging is the "Rule of Thirds." This rule suggests we should only take one-third when encountering a patch of the desired plant. One-third is left to continue the plant's life cycle and maintain the population's health, and another third is left for wildlife that may also depend on the plant for food, shelter, or other needs. This rule is needed so that we do not deplete the plant populations or disrupt the larger ecosystem.

Another fundamental tenet of ethical foraging is gaining appropriate knowledge about the plants we want to gather. This includes correctly identifying the plant and knowing the best time to harvest for optimal potency. A good forager will also be aware of the plant's conservation status. Some plants are endangered or threatened, and these should never be harvested from the wild. Instead, efforts can be made to cultivate such plants at home or source them from reputable suppliers who practice sustainable cultivation.

Before heading out to forage, it's also crucial to be aware of and respect property boundaries and regulations. Always ask permission if you plan to forage on private land, and familiarize yourself with the rules and restrictions if you plan to forage in public areas like parks or national forests.

Furthermore, consider the environment's health where the plants are growing. Avoid gathering plants from polluted areas or places exposed to heavy pesticide use, as these contaminants can accumulate in the plants and be harmful to ingest.

Ethical foraging calls for gratitude, a heartfelt thankfulness to nature for its generous gifts. Some people express this gratitude by saying a few words of thanks; others might leave a small offering or simply take a moment to acknowledge the exchange. This act of gratitude completes the circle of giving and receiving, reminding us of our interconnectedness with nature and all life.

The Evolving Role of Herbalists

In a fortunate turn of events, the role of herbalists in the future of herbal medicine is evolving and expanding. No longer confined to the margins of healthcare, herbalists are actively collaborating with conventional healthcare practitioners, working in integrative medical settings, and offering their expertise to a broader audience.

For instance, herbalists may work alongside doctors and nurses in integrative clinics, providing patients with herbal consultations and personalized recommendations. This collaborative approach benefits the patients and helps bridge the gap between conventional medicine and herbalism, fostering a greater understanding and appreciation for the value of plant-based healing.

Key Reasons to Consider Natural Remedies

As people are increasingly seeking alternatives or complementary therapies to address their health concerns, herbal remedies have become more popular and effective. Here are some key reasons why herbal remedies are game-changers in today's world:

- Natural and holistic approach: Herbal remedies provide a natural and holistic way to treat various health issues, working harmoniously with the body's biological healing processes. This approach often focuses on addressing the root cause of a problem rather than just alleviating symptoms, promoting overall health and well-being.

- Prevention and maintenance: Herbal remedies can prevent health issues, strengthen the immune system, and maintain good health. By incorporating herbs into one's daily routine, individuals can support their body's natural defenses and promote overall wellness.

- Complementary therapy: Herbal medicine can be used alongside conventional medical treatments, enhancing their effectiveness and potentially reducing side effects. For example, herbs like ginger and peppermint can help alleviate nausea associated with chemotherapy, while St. John's Wort can be an effective supplement for managing mild to moderate depression.

- Lower risk of side effects: Herbal remedies generally have fewer side effects than synthetic drugs, which makes them a safer option for many individuals. However, it is essential to use herbs responsibly and under the guidance of a qualified healthcare professional, as some herbs may interact with medications or cause adverse reactions in some individuals.

- Accessible and affordable: Herbal remedies can be more affordable and accessible than conventional medications, particularly in areas where access to healthcare may be limited. Using local plants and herbs can provide cost-effective alternatives for managing common health issues.

- Preservation of traditional knowledge: The use of herbal remedies helps preserve traditional knowledge and cultural practices passed down through generations. This wealth of knowledge has been accumulated over thousands of years and forms an essential part of our global heritage.

- Sustainable healthcare: Using herbal remedies supports sustainable healthcare practices, reducing reliance on synthetic drugs and promoting environmental conservation. By cultivating and using local plants, communities can reduce their ecological footprint and contribute to biodiversity.

Safety and Precautions

A common misconception is that utilizing plants for medicinal purposes is inherently safer than using pharmaceutical drugs. Given the extensive heritage of plant-based folk medicine, it is no surprise that this concept has gained considerable popularity. However, "natural" is NOT synonymous with safety. When not used correctly, some herbal remedies can have unfavorable reactions with other medications or become toxic at high doses, causing side effects.

To provide you with a heads-up regarding the interactions between herbal remedies and conventional medications or drugs, here are some examples:

- Kava, an herb traditionally used to address anxiety, insomnia, menopause symptoms, and other conditions, has shown promise in alleviating stress. However, it can lead to severe liver damage, prompting the FDA to warn against its use.

- St. John's Wort may be effective for mild to moderate depression but can interfere with birth control pills, antidepressants, and other medications. Additionally, it may cause side effects like stomach discomfort and anxiety.

- Yohimbe, a bark utilized for treating erectile dysfunction, can result in high blood pressure, increased heart rate, anxiety, and other adverse effects. It can also interact with certain antidepressants. Using it in high doses or for an extended period can be hazardous.

The term "natural" is not a reliable indicator of which herbal treatments are safe and which pose potential risks. To ensure that you reap the benefits of herbal medicine while minimizing potential harm, consider the following safety tips and precautions:

1. Ask an expert in the field: Before starting any new herbal remedy, consult a healthcare professional or a qualified herbalist. They can help guide you toward the most appropriate herbs for your specific health concerns and advise you on the correct dosage and duration of use.

2. Be aware of potential interactions: Certain herbs can interact with prescription medications or other herbs, leading to potentially harmful effects. For instance, ginkgo biloba may interact with the blood thinner Warfarin, increasing the risk of excessive bleeding. Always consult with your healthcare provider about any herbal remedies you are incorporating to prevent adverse interactions.

3. Quality matters: Choose high-quality herbal products from reputable manufacturers. Low-quality or adulterated products may not provide the desired benefits and may even pose risks to your health. Look for standardized extracts, which guarantee a consistent level of the active ingredients in the product.

4. Follow recommended dosages: Adherence to the recommended dosages for herbal remedies is fundamental, as excessive consumption can lead to unwanted side effects. Remember that more is

not always better, and exceeding the suggested dosage can sometimes be harmful.

5. Be cautious with self-diagnosis: While it may be tempting and comfortable to self-diagnose and self-treat, you must always seek professional guidance when dealing with health issues, particularly for severe or persistent symptoms. Misdiagnosing and treating a condition with the wrong herbal remedy can be counterproductive and potentially harmful.

6. Allergies and sensitivities: Watch out for potential allergies or sensitivities to certain herbs, particularly if you have a history of allergies to plants, pollen, or other natural substances. Start with a small dose and observe for any adverse reactions before increasing the dosage.

7. Special populations: Pregnant and breastfeeding women, children, and older adults should exercise special caution when using herbal remedies. Some herbs may contain substances that can be harmful to these sensitive populations and should only be used under the careful supervision of a healthcare professional.

By following these safety precautions and consulting with a qualified healthcare professional, you can safely and effectively incorporate herbal remedies into your wellness routine.

Chapter Two
Understanding Herbs and Their Benefits

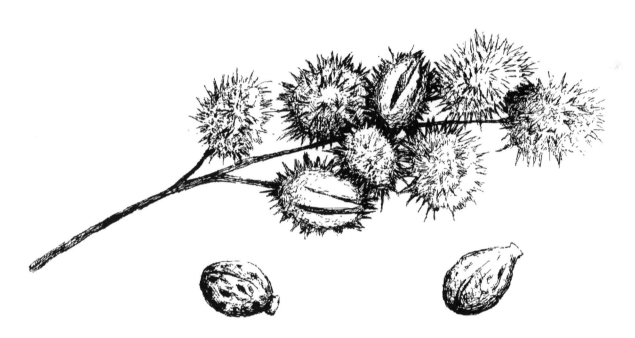

Throughout this chapter, we'll learn about the science behind how herbs work, the various active ingredients that give them their unique properties, and the differences and synergies between herbal remedies and conventional medicine. So, buckle up and get ready for an exciting journey to better understand the incredible world of herbs and their benefits!

How Herbs Work in the Body

Phytochemicals are a diverse group of naturally occurring compounds found in plants, which play an essential role in their growth, protection, and overall vitality. These potent compounds, also called plant secondary metabolites, give plants their distinctive colors, flavors, and aromas, offering various health-promoting benefits when consumed by humans.

There are thousands of known phytochemicals, such as flavonoids, carotenoids, alkaloids, and terpenes, each with unique properties and potential health benefits. For example, flavonoids are known for their antioxidant and anti-inflammatory effects, while alkaloids can have stimulant or analgesic properties.

The synergistic effect of multiple compounds

Unlike conventional medications, which typically contain isolated active ingredients, herbal remedies offer a unique approach; that is, they consist of a blend of natural compounds called phytochemicals, each with its own therapeutic properties. These phytochemicals interact synergistically, creating a combined effect surpassing their actions' sum. This phenomenon, known as synergy, allows herbal medicine to harness the full potential of the diverse phytochemicals present in a single plant or a combination of plants. By working together, these compounds enhance the overall therapeutic benefits and promote a more holistic approach to healing.

For example, the anti-inflammatory properties of turmeric are mainly attributed to its primary active compound, curcumin. However, when combined with other phytochemicals in the turmeric plant or with compounds found in black pepper, such as piperine, curcumin's bioavailability and efficacy are significantly increased.

This synergistic effect is an essential aspect of herbal medicine, as it allows for a more comprehensive approach to healing that considers the complex interplay of various compounds, ultimately leading to more effective and well-rounded treatment options.

Herbs provide therapeutic benefits through their special effects on various systems in the body, which are referred to as "herbal actions." These actions are categorized as adaptogens, nervines, carminatives, or diuretics, and each has a distinct impact on the body's systems.

Herbal Actions and Their Effects on Bodily Systems

For example, adaptogens are a class of herbs that, by balancing hormones and regulating the adrenal system, assist the body in adapting to physical, mental, and emotional stress. Ginseng (Panax ginseng), a well-known adaptogen, has been used for ages to boost energy, lessen weariness, and enhance general well-being.

On the other side, nervene herbs work on the nervous system and can aid in reducing stress, tension, and anxiety. Chamomile (Matricaria chamomilla), a well-liked nervine, is frequently consumed as a soothing herbal tea to reduce stress and encourage sound sleep.

Choosing the right herbs to address specific needs and health conditions requires understanding the numerous herbal activities and their effects on various biological systems. Herbalists can design efficient treatment regimens that support the body's natural healing processes and advance general health and well-being by focusing herbal remedies on the underlying imbalances in the body.

The Influence of Herbs on the Body's Natural Healing Processes

In my professional experience, I have seen many situations where herbs have helped support the body's natural healing processes. Herbs can improve the body's innate ability to restore balance and promote overall well-being by working harmoniously with its various systems.

I will never forget a client suffering from chronic digestive issues. Despite using a variety of traditional treatments, he could not achieve long-term relief. Following a thorough consultation, I prescribed a blend of herbs recognized for their relaxing and digestive-supportive characteristics, including marshmallow root, slippery elm, and fennel.

Over time, the client noticed a significant improvement in his symptoms, as the herbal blend helped to reduce inflammation, soothe irritation, and promote healthy digestion. This not only treated his immediate difficulties, but it also improved his overall health by assisting the body's natural healing processes.

This holistic approach underlines the importance of treating the underlying imbalances rather than merely suppressing symptoms, allowing for long-term wellness. By providing gentle and targeted support, herbs effectively promote optimal health while minimizing the risk of unwanted side effects often associated with conventional treatments.

Active Ingredients in Herbs

This section will look at five different types of active compounds: alkaloids, flavonoids, essential oils, tannins, and saponins. Each of these groupings provides distinct advantages, ranging from antioxidant effects to immune-boosting characteristics, and understanding their roles in herbal medicine can help us appreciate the power of plants.

Alkaloids and their medicinal properties

Alkaloids are a group of naturally occurring organic compounds found in many herbs and plants, characterized by their nitrogen-containing structure. These potent compounds often have significant medicinal properties, which makes them essential to herbal medicine.

I have personally witnessed the extraordinary effectiveness of alkaloids on various health problems. The poppy plant (Papaver somniferum), which contains morphine and codeine, both potent pain relievers, is one of the most well-known examples of an alkaloid-rich botanical. While these components have been extracted and utilized in traditional pain treatments, other alkaloids and phytochemicals in the poppy plant provide additional benefits.

Another example is the alkaloid berberine, found in herbs such as goldenseal (Hydrastis canadensis) and barberry (Berberis vulgaris). Berberine has demonstrated antimicrobial, anti-inflammatory, and blood sugar-lowering effects, making it a valuable herbal remedy for various health issues, including digestive problems and type 2 diabetes.

The wide variety of alkaloids found in herbs plays a significant role in their therapeutic properties, providing numerous healing benefits that can be utilized in herbal medicine.

Flavonoids and Their Antioxidant Effects

Flavonoids are a diverse group of plant compounds known for their vibrant colors and powerful antioxidant properties. These natural substances are abundant in many fruits, vegetables, and herbs, providing not only visual allure but also a multitude of health benefits.

Whenever I discuss flavonoids, my excitement grows as I am always fascinated by how incredibly these compounds can improve our health. As I said, the most notable aspect is their antioxidant properties, helping to counteract harmful free radicals, which are unstable molecules that can cause damage to our cells and contribute to chronic diseases and aging. It's incredible to see how flavonoids can play a vital role in protecting our well-being. Isn't it?

Do you want to know about one of my favorite herbs rich in flavonoids? It is called hawthorn (or Crataegus), which has been used traditionally to support heart health. The flavonoids found in hawthorn berries, leaves, and flowers improve circulation, strengthen blood vessels, and even lower blood pressure. I have witnessed clients experiencing significant improvements in their cardiovascular health after incorporating hawthorn into their wellness routines.

Another example? The well-known green tea (Camellia sinensis) is packed with a type of flavonoid called catechins. These potent antioxidants have been shown to support healthy metabolism, protect against cellular damage, and even reduce the risk of certain types of cancer.

Essential oils and their aromatic benefits

Essential oils, which are highly concentrated aromatic compounds found in herbs and plants, have a long history of being used for healing purposes. These volatile oils can be extracted from various plant parts, such as flowers, leaves, bark, or roots, and are responsible for the characteristic scents of many herbs.

I remember a client struggling with sleep and anxiety for over a year. I suggested incorporating lavender (Lavandula angustifolia) essential oil into their bedtime routine, as it has a well-documented calming effect on the nervous system. The client started using a diffuser with a few drops of lavender oil in their bedroom each night and soon noticed a significant improvement in their sleep quality and overall relaxation.

In addition to lavender, there are other essential oils that have a wide range of aromatic benefits. For instance, peppermint (Mentha Piperita) essential oil is known for its invigorating and refreshing scent, which can help boost energy and mental clarity. On the other hand, rosemary (Rosmarinus officinalis) essential oil has been shown to enhance memory and cognitive function, making it an excellent aid for focus and concentration.

The aromatic qualities of essential oils go beyond their pleasant scents, providing healing effects that extend to both the body and the mind.

Tannins and their astringent properties

Tannins are a group of naturally occurring plant compounds with astringent properties, which means they can cause the contraction of skin and mucous membranes. Because of this distinguishing feature, tannins are helpful in herbal medicine for treating ailments such as inflammation, bleeding, and skin irritations.

Witch hazel (Hamamelis virginiana) is an example of a tannin-rich herb. This herb is famous for its astringent and anti-inflammatory properties, which make it an effective treatment for skin conditions such as acne, eczema, and even hemorrhoids. Witch hazel extract is a key ingredient in many over-the-counter skin care treatments for reducing redness, swelling, and pore size.

Also, Black tea (Camellia sinensis) includes a high level of tannins, contributing to its characteristic flavor and dark color. Because black tea's astringent characteristics can soothe inflamed tissues, it's a popular home cure for sunburns, puffy eyes, and minor cuts or scrapes.

Saponins and their immune-boosting effects

Saponins are natural organic compounds that generate soapy lathers when mixed with water. Beyond their foaming properties, saponins have been shown to exhibit a range of health benefits, including immune-boosting effects that make them valuable in herbal medicine.

Astragalus (Astragalus membranaceus), a well-known saponin-rich herb, is a staple in traditional Chinese medicine. Because of its high saponin content, astragalus has been utilized to strengthen the immune system for ages.

Another example is Echinacea, a popular immune-boosting herb native to North America. Echinacea's saponins contribute to its ability to activate the immune system, which aids in the prevention of colds, flu, and other illnesses. During the cold and flu season, many people use echinacea supplements to boost their immune system and minimize the severity of their condition.

Herbal Remedies vs. Conventional Medicine

As an herbalist, I often converse about the differences and similarities between herbal remedies and conventional medicine. While both approaches have unique advantages and challenges, they can also work together to create a more comprehensive approach to health.

- Source of Treatments - Herbal remedies rely on the healing properties of plants, using various plant parts like leaves, roots, flowers, and seeds. Conversely, conventional medicine often involves synthetic or chemically derived drugs typically formulated in labs.

- Interaction with the Body - Herbal remedies work more gently and harmoniously with the body's natural processes, while conventional drugs can sometimes have more targeted and potent effects. However, this also means that herbal remedies may take longer to show results, whereas traditional medicines often provide more immediate relief.

- Side Effects and Safety - Herbal remedies generally have fewer side effects and a lower dependency risk than conventional medications. However, this doesn't mean that herbal remedies are without risk. Remember that herbs can still interact with other medicines, and it's essential to consult a healthcare professional before starting any new herbal regimen.

- Standardization and Dosage - Conventional medicine typically offers a higher degree of standardization in terms of dosage and potency. Herbal remedies can vary in strength and composition, depending on factors such as growing conditions, harvesting methods, and preparation techniques. Practitioners and consumers must know their herbs and use reliable sources to assure quality and safety.

- Integrative Approach - Despite their differences, herbal remedies and conventional medicine can complement each other when used together in an integrative approach. For example, I've seen people find relief from pain by combining herbal anti-inflammatory remedies like turmeric (Curcuma longa) with conventional pain relievers or by using adaptogenic herbs like Ashwagandha (Withania somnifera) to help manage the side effects of prescription medications.

Ultimately, the choice between herbal and conventional medicine is personal, often influenced by personal beliefs, individual needs, and the specific health concern being addressed. It is essential to consult with healthcare professionals, who can provide guidance and help navigate the options to determine the most appropriate and effective course of treatment for each individual.

Chapter Three

Integrating Herbal Remedies Into Your Lifestyle

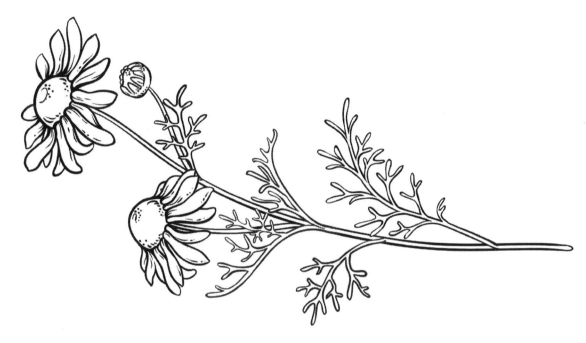

Herbal remedies come in various forms, each with its unique characteristics. Choosing the right form basically depends on several factors, including the type of herb, its taste, the desired effect, the ease of use, and individual preferences.

For example, someone with a busy schedule might prefer capsules or tinctures because they are easy to take and require no preparation time. In contrast, someone who enjoys the ritual of preparing their remedies might prefer teas or infusions. Similarly, topical application would be the best choice if the goal is to treat a skin condition. Therefore, it is essential to understand the characteristics of each form to make an informed decision.

Powdered Form

Powdered herbal remedies are dried herbs that have been ground into a fine dust. But what makes them so fascinating is their incredible versatility. How would you like to incorporate powdered herbs into your daily routine? There are many ways to do so: perhaps mixing them into your favorite foods or drinks, encapsulating them for easy consumption, or even experimenting with making herbal pastes. Some people even add powdered herbs to bathwater for a soothing, therapeutic soak.

One of the primary advantages of powdered herbs is that they are typically easy to digest, and the body can quickly absorb their therapeutic components; that's why they can also be mixed into almost any food or drink, allowing you to easily incorporate them into your diet. However, not all herbs are for everyone; some powdered herbs can have a strong taste that some might find unpleasant. Also, they can be slightly messy, and measuring out precise dosages can sometimes be tricky.

When it comes to storage, powdered herbs should be kept in a cool, dry place away from sunlight. An airtight container is ideal as it prevents moisture from getting in, which could lead to mold growth. Some people prefer storing powdered herbs in the refrigerator to extend their shelf life. As for usage, follow the recommended dosage provided on the packaging or advised by a healthcare professional. You might start with a small amount to see how your body reacts and then adjust the dosage as needed.

For example, suppose you're adding powdered turmeric to your smoothie for its anti-inflammatory benefits. In that case, you might start with a quarter teaspoon and then gradually increase to a full teaspoon if you find it beneficial and tolerable.

Capsules and Tablets

Capsules and tablets are familiar forms of herbal remedies, offering convenience and ease of use. Herbal capsules are small, cylindrical containers typically made of gelatin or a vegan equivalent. These capsules are filled with powdered herbs. Tablets, on the other hand, are compressed powdered herbs formed into solid, usually round or oblong shapes. Both capsules and tablets are designed for oral consumption, and their size makes them easy to swallow.

When it comes to capsules and tablets, convenience is the name of the game. They are portable, easy to take, and require no preparation time. Additionally, they mask the taste of the herb, which can be beneficial when consuming herbs with strong or bitter flavors. One potential downside is that capsules and tablets might take longer to digest and absorb than other forms like tinctures or powders. Also, it can be challenging to adjust the dosage with capsules and tablets because they come in pre-measured amounts.

When using capsules or tablets, follow the recommended dosage instructions on the product label or as advised by a healthcare professional. Generally, they are taken with a glass of water to ease swallowing and digestion. Remember that the potency of herbal remedies can vary from one product to another, so it's crucial to start with a low dose and gradually increase as needed. Store capsules and tablets in a cool, dry place, away from direct sunlight, and close the bottle tightly after each use to maintain their potency.

Tinctures and Liquid Extracts

Tinctures and liquid extracts are concentrated herbal remedies prepared by soaking herbs in a mixture of water and alcohol or glycerin. The process extracts the herb's therapeutic properties, producing a powerful liquid solution. Tinctures should be stored in small glass bottles with a dropper for easy administration.

Tinctures and liquid extracts offer several advantages. Their highly concentrated nature means only a small amount can unleash their therapeutic effects. The liquid form allows quick absorption into the bloodstream, often leading to faster results than other forms like capsules or tablets. Furthermore, the dosage can be easily adjusted, making tinctures suitable for individualized treatment plans. On the downside, the taste of some tinctures can be pretty strong due to the alcohol content, and they may not be suitable for individuals who need to avoid alcohol.

Regarding dosage and administration, tinctures are typically taken orally, either directly under the tongue (sublingually) or diluted in a small amount of water or juice. The sublingual method allows the tincture to be absorbed directly into the bloodstream, bypassing the digestive system for a quicker effect. Dosage varies widely depending on the type of herb and the individual's health condition, but a common starting point might be a few drops to a full dropper taken 1-3 times per day.

Always follow the specific dosage instructions provided on the label or advised by a healthcare professional. To store tinctures, keep them in a cool, dark place, like a cupboard or pantry, and always ensure the cap is tightly sealed after use to maintain potency.

Herbal Teas and Infusions

Herbal teas and infusions are beverages made by steeping herbs, flowers, seeds, or roots in hot water. This process allows the water to absorb the plant's beneficial compounds, creating a therapeutic drink. This category has two main types of herbal preparations: infusions and decoctions. Infusions involve steeping delicate parts of the plant, like leaves or flowers, whereas decoctions require boiling tougher parts, like roots or bark.

Herbal teas and infusions are quite versatile. They can be enjoyed hot or cold, and their flavors can be enhanced with natural sweeteners like honey or stevia. Additionally, preparing and drinking herbal tea can be a relaxing ritual, adding a mental wellness aspect to their physical benefits. However, herbal teas and infusions may take longer to prepare than other herbal remedies, and the taste might not appeal to everyone.

When it comes to brewing, the general guideline for making an infusion is to use one teaspoon of dried herb or two teaspoons of fresh herb per cup of boiling water. Allow the mixture to steep for 10-15 minutes, then strain the herbs before drinking. For a decoction, simmer the herbs in water for approximately 15-20 minutes before straining.

How to maximize the benefits of your infusions

1. Source High-Quality Herbs

The quality of your infusion depends mainly on the quality of the herbs you use. Always source the best quality herbs you can find. Look for organic herbs, which will be free from harmful pesticides and other chemicals. Fresh herbs often provide the best flavor and the highest concentration of beneficial compounds, but dried herbs can also be effective and are more convenient for many people. Whether fresh or dried, the herbs should be vibrant in color and have a strong aroma, as these are indications of good quality.

2. Use the Correct Water Temperature

The temperature at which you steep your herbs can significantly impact the efficacy of your infusion. Some delicate herbs may lose their beneficial compounds if the water is too hot, while tougher, woody herbs might require a higher temperature to fully release their properties. Generally, use boiling water (212°F or 100°C) for tougher, woody herbs like roots, barks, and seeds. For more delicate herbs, like leaves and flowers, use water that is near boiling (185°F to 205°F or 85°C to 95°C).

3. Pay Attention to Steep Time

Just as the water temperature is important, so is the steep time. Steep your herbs long enough to extract the beneficial compounds but not so long that the infusion becomes bitter and unpalatable. Generally, a steep time of 10-15 minutes is appropriate for most herbs, but you may need to adjust this depending on the specific herbs you're using and your taste preferences.

4. Cover Your Infusion While Steeping

During the steeping process, your infusion will be releasing volatile compounds - these are often the components with the most health benefits, as well as the most flavor and aroma. While the herbs are steeping, cap your mug or teapot to prevent the chemical compounds from evaporating into the air.

5. Measure Properly

While eyeballing amounts may seem more straightforward, proper measurement can go a long way in ensuring the effectiveness of your herbal infusion. Too few herbs might result in a weak infusion that doesn't provide the desired health benefits. Too many herbs could result in an overly strong, bitter taste and might even cause side effects if the herbs are particularly potent. As a general guideline, use one tablespoon of dried herbs or two tablespoons of fresh herbs for each cup of water.

6. Consume Infusions Promptly

The effectiveness of herbal infusions can diminish or even fade over time, even when properly stored. Many of the most beneficial compounds in herbs are volatile, meaning they will gradually evaporate at room temperature. Aim to consume it soon after it has finished steeping to get the most benefit from your infusion.

While refrigeration can help preserve the potency of an infusion if you can't consume it immediately, even in the fridge, the volatile compounds can slowly evaporate. So as a general rule, the fresher the infusion, the better. Make your infusions when you have the time to consume the drink immediately and appreciate the fresh, vibrant flavors and maximum health benefits that your herbs may offer.

Topical Applications

Topical herbal remedies are designed for external use and come in various forms, such as ointments, creams, balms, salves, and oils. These remedies are typically made by infusing herbs into a base like oil or wax. The resulting product is applied directly to the skin to address various issues, from minor cuts and burns to more complex skin conditions like eczema or psoriasis.

One major advantage of topical applications is their ability to target specific areas. If you're dealing with a localized issue like a wound or a rash, applying an herbal remedy directly to the problem area can give you quick and effective relief.

Moreover, because they're used externally, topical remedies bypass the digestive system, reducing the risk of systemic side effects. However, these remedies may not be suitable for all skin types. Some individuals might experience skin irritation or allergic reactions to certain ingredients. Therefore, it's always a good idea to do a patch test on a small skin area before full application.

When using a topical herbal remedy, clean the application area first to prevent any dirt or bacteria from being trapped under the product. Apply a small amount of the product to the affected area, following any specific instructions on the packaging. For instance, some products may advise against applying on broken skin or near the eyes.

In general, less is more when it comes to topical applications - a thin layer is usually sufficient. After applying, allow the product to absorb fully into the skin. Store your topical remedies in a cool, dry place, away from direct sunlight. Of course, if you notice any discomfort or adverse reactions like redness, itchiness, or swelling, discontinue use and consult a healthcare professional.

Other Forms

Besides the forms discussed so far, herbal remedies also come in other forms as well, such as poultices, syrups, and inhalants, each offering unique benefits.

Poultices are a kind of herbal paste made by crushing fresh or dried herbs and mixing them with a little water. This paste is then applied directly to the skin, often with a cloth or bandage, to address localized issues like wounds, sprains, or skin inflammations. They offer a concentrated dose of the herb's therapeutic compounds where required.

Syrups, on the other hand, are sweetened, concentrated herbal infusions. They're typically used for treating throat or respiratory issues. Elderberry syrup, for example, is a popular remedy for cold and flu symptoms. The sweet taste of syrups makes them particularly suitable for children who might find other forms of herbal remedies less palatable.

Inhalants are another herbal remedy that involves breathing in the therapeutic aroma of herbs, usually through steam. This can be particularly beneficial for respiratory issues, relaxation, and stress relief.

Considerations and uses for these forms include:

- Poultices: Ideal for localized skin issues or injuries; always test a small area first to ensure there's no adverse reaction.

- Syrups: Useful for soothing sore throats or coughs; always check for potential allergens, especially if given to children.

- Inhalants: Excellent for respiratory issues or relaxation; use caution with the temperature of the steam to avoid burns.

Factors to Consider When Choosing a Form

What factors do you find most important when choosing an herbal remedy? Is it the convenience, versatility, or simplicity that resonates with you the most? Picking the right form of herbal remedy is a nuanced process, often hinging on several factors. As an herbalist with years of professional experience, I've seen first-hand how personal preferences and convenience can strongly influence this choice. For example, if you're often on the go, you might prefer capsules or tablets due to their portability and ease of use. Conversely, herbal infusions might be your go-to if you enjoy the ritualistic aspect of brewing a soothing cup of tea.

A second key factor is bioavailability and absorption - how quickly and efficiently your body can absorb the beneficial compounds in the herb. Tinctures and liquid extracts, for instance, are rapidly absorbed when taken sublingually, making them an excellent choice if you're seeking quick relief.

The form you choose might also depend on the specific health conditions and target areas you're addressing. Topical applications like creams and ointments are often best for skin-related issues, while syrups might be chosen for respiratory or throat ailments.

Lastly, consider the dosage and potency requirements. Concentrating forms like tinctures or capsules might be the most effective if you need a high-potency remedy.

Here are a few questions that might guide your decision:

- What is your daily routine like? Do you need something easy and quick, or enjoy a slow, ritualistic process?

- What are your health goals? Are you targeting a specific area or seeking general wellness?

- Are you comfortable with intense flavors, or would you prefer something tasteless?

- Do you need to adjust your dosage frequently, or is a standard dosage sufficient for your needs?

Remember, what works best for one person might not be the best choice for another. It's a highly personal process, so feel free to experiment and see what works best for you.

Personal Preferences and Convenience

Personal preferences and lifestyle considerations can largely influence the decision to choose a particular form of herbal remedy. For instance, if you enjoy rituals and the slow unfolding of experiences, preparing and sipping on a warm cup of herbal tea might fascinate you. The act of brewing the tea not only offers therapeutic benefits but can also serve as a calming ritual that anchors your day.

On the other hand, if your days are packed and you're always on the move, convenience might be your top priority. In this case, herbal capsules or tablets are a perfect fit. They can easily be carried in a bag or pocket and consumed quickly without any preparation. No need to worry about steeping times or boiling water - just a quick sip, and you're good to go!

If you're not a fan of strong or bitter herbal flavors, capsules and tablets can change the game for you. They encapsulate the herbal material, effectively masking any off-putting tastes. In contrast, if you're a flavor enthusiast who loves exploring unique taste profiles, experimenting with different herbal teas and tinctures could be an exciting journey.

The most effective form of herbal remedy is the one you're comfortable with and fits seamlessly into your lifestyle. It's about finding that sweet spot where convenience meets preference, transforming your path to wellness into an enjoyable journey rather than a tedious chore.

Bioavailability and absorption

Bioavailability refers to the amount and rate at which a substance is absorbed into your bloodstream. Regarding herbal remedies, different forms can have different levels of bioavailability. Understanding this can help you choose the form that best fits your needs.

For example, tinctures and liquid extracts are known for their high bioavailability. These are typically taken sublingually or under the tongue, where the rich network of blood vessels allows for rapid absorption directly into the bloodstream. This quick action can be especially beneficial when swift relief is needed, such as for the sudden onset of a headache or a bout of insomnia.

Capsules and tablets, while convenient and easy to use, may have lower bioavailability. They must first pass through the digestive system before the beneficial compounds are released and absorbed, which can take some time. However, the gradual release of the herbal constituents can provide sustained benefits over a longer period.

Herbal teas and infusions sit somewhere in between. The hot water extraction process releases the beneficial compounds absorbed as you drink the tea. This method offers both the herbs' therapeutic benefits and water's hydration benefits.

Here's a quick rundown:

- Tinctures and liquid extracts: High bioavailability, fast absorption.

- Capsules and tablets: Lower bioavailability, gradual release.

- Herbal teas and infusions: Moderate bioavailability, added hydration benefits.

Choosing a form based on its bioavailability and absorption is all about aligning the remedy with your health needs. A quick-acting tincture might be suitable for sudden symptoms, while a slow-release capsule could be the best bet for ongoing support.

Specific health conditions and target areas

The specific health condition you aim to address, and the target area can significantly influence the choice of herbal remedy form. Each form has its strengths when addressing specific issues or areas of the body.

For example, if you're dealing with a skin issue like a rash or a minor wound, a topical form like a cream, salve, or ointment could be your best bet. These are applied directly to the skin, enabling the herbs' therapeutic ingredients to operate instantly where they are most needed.

An herbal syrup could be the answer to soothe a sore throat or a cough. The thick, sweet liquid can coat the throat, relieving irritation. On the other hand, if you're dealing with a digestive issue, capsules or tablets could be a good option, as they release their beneficial compounds in the gut, where they can have the most effect.

For stress relief or sleep support, consider an herbal tea or infusion. The act of sipping a warm drink can be calming in itself, while the beneficial compounds in the herbs can help to relax the mind and body.

Dosage and potency requirements

Different forms of herbal remedies offer varying levels of potency, and understanding this can guide your selection process.

Capsules and tablets, for instance, typically contain a standardized amount of the active constituents of an herb. They can offer a high level of potency and consistency in dosage, which can be especially useful for conditions requiring a precise amount of the herb. For example, if a healthcare professional recommends a specific St. John's Wort dosage for mood support, capsules or tablets could be the most reliable way to ensure you get the required amount.

Tinctures and liquid extracts, on the other hand, are highly concentrated and deliver a high degree of efficacy. They come with a dropper for easy dosage adjustments. This can be especially useful if you're new to a particular herb and want to start with a smaller dose and gradually increase it as needed.

Herbal teas and infusions offer the lowest potency compared to other forms. The beneficial compounds are diluted in water; not all compounds may be water-soluble. However, the lower potency doesn't mean they're ineffective. A cup of chamomile tea before bedtime, for example, can be just the thing to gently soothe and prepare you for sleep.

In summary:

- Capsules and tablets: High potency, consistent dosage, good for specific dosage requirements.

- Tinctures and liquid extracts: High potency, adjustable dosage, suitable for a gradual dose increase.

- Herbal teas and infusions: Lower potency, good for gentle, supportive effects.

Choosing the proper form based on dosage and potency requirements is about finding a balance between effectiveness and your comfort level with the herb.

BOOK II

HERBAL REMEDIES FOR COMMON AILMENTS

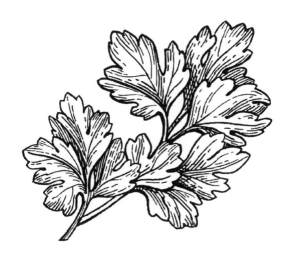

AMBER WHITMORE

Introduction

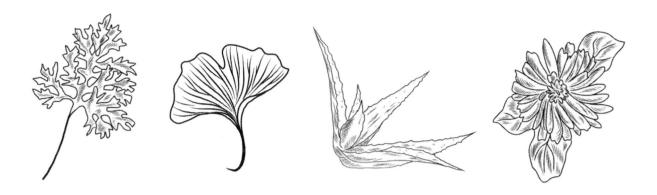

As we move into the world of herbal remedies for common ailments, we need to know that each person's journey with herbal medicine is unique. What works for one person may not work for another, and finding the right combination of herbs and lifestyle adjustments often requires patience, experimentation, and self-awareness. With that in mind, I'm excited to share my insights as an herbalist to help guide you through the fascinating world of plant-based healing.

Here, we will explore different herbs and natural remedies to address common health concerns that many of us face in our daily lives. From allergies and asthma to stress and sleep disorders, we'll discuss the healing potential of plants and how they can help support our overall well-being.

As someone who has personally witnessed the remarkable impact of herbs in addressing my own health concerns and those of my clients, I can attest to the profound difference these natural remedies can make. Whether it's the soothing properties of chamomile (Matricaria chamomilla) for a racing mind or the immune-boosting benefits of Echinacea (Echinacea spp.) during cold and flu season, the wisdom of plants has become an inseparable part of my health journey and that of countless others.

Now let's discover how herbs and remedies can help alleviate our ailments, offering practical suggestions to help us make thoughtful decisions about our health.

Chapter One
Common Conditions

Allergies and Asthma

Allergies and asthma are widespread health issues affecting millions of individuals around the world. Allergies develop when the immune system reacts abnormally to an innocuous element, such as pollen, pet dander, or specific foods.

This immunological reaction can result in various symptoms, such as sneezing, itching, and congestion. Asthma, however, is a chronic inflammatory disease that affects the airways and causes symptoms such as wheezing, shortness of breath, and chest tightness. Allergies and asthma can substantially impact a person's quality of life, so finding effective strategies to control and alleviate these symptoms is critical.

Herbal medicines can help control allergies and asthma naturally, alongside conventional therapies or as stand-alone choices for milder symptoms. Some herbs can aid in reducing inflammation, soothing inflamed airways, and the immune system's response to allergens.

Mullein

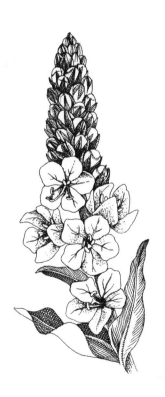

Mullein, scientifically called Verbascum thapsus, is recognized in herbal medicine for its potential to treat respiratory issues. This plant's potent properties provide a natural alternative for those suffering from allergies and asthma.

The magic of mullein resides primarily in its leaves and flowers. These parts of the plant are a rich source of compounds that can help alleviate inflammation in the respiratory tract. This anti-inflammatory effect can be especially beneficial for individuals with allergies, as it may reduce the discomfort caused by inflamed nasal and throat tissues. For asthmatics, this reduction in inflammation can facilitate easier breathing and decrease the severity of asthma attacks.

Moreover, mullein has a gentle expectorant characteristic, which aids in loosening and removing mucus from the airways. This property can benefit those dealing with congestion due to allergies or asthma. Clearing mucus build-up, mullein can promote better airflow and improves respiratory function.

Mullein can be consumed in various ways to reap its respiratory benefits. For instance, the dried leaves and flowers can be steeped to create a soothing tea. The plant can also be transformed into a tincture, a concentrated herbal extract. This tincture can be mixed with water or juice for consumption. Alternatively, mullein can be encapsulated and taken as a dietary supplement. This flexibility in preparation methods enables individuals to choose the method that works best for their lifestyle and personal preferences.

While mullein is cultivated in various parts of the world for its medicinal uses, it also grows naturally in many places. It's easily recognizable with its tall, erect stem that can grow up to 2 meters high and its large, woolly leaves. It thrives predominantly in uncultivated, dry soils, fields, roadsides, or waste grounds. It's a biennial plant, completing its life cycle in two years. It produces a spike of yellow flowers used medicinally during its second year.

Nettle

Stinging nettle (Urtica dioica) is a perennial plant commonly found in various parts of the world. Known for its irritating hairs on its leaves and stems, this plant may cause discomfort upon contact. However, when prepared and appropriately consumed, stinging nettle offers a range of health benefits, particularly for those suffering from allergies and asthma.

One of the primary benefits of stinging nettle is its natural antihistamine and anti-inflammatory compounds. These properties can help alleviate allergy symptoms such as:

- Nasal congestion

- Sneezing

- Itching

- Watery eyes

By inhibiting the release of histamines, which are the main cause of allergy symptoms, stinging nettle can relieve those suffering from seasonal allergies or hay fever.

Stinging nettle may also help reduce inflammation in the airways, which can be particularly beneficial for individuals with asthma. By minimizing inflammation, it can potentially improve breathing and lessen the severity of asthma attacks.

There are several ways to consume stinging nettle for its health benefits:

1. Tea: Nettle leaves can be steeped in hot water to create a soothing herbal tea. To make nettle tea, add 1-2 teaspoons of dried nettle leaves to a cup of boiling water, let it steep for about 10 minutes, and then strain the leaves before drinking.

2. Tincture: Nettle tinctures are concentrated liquid extracts that can be purchased or made at home. To use a nettle tincture, add a few drops to a glass of water and consume as directed on the label.

3. Capsules: Nettle supplements are available in capsule form and can be taken as directed on the label. These capsules often contain a blend of nettle and other beneficial herbs, such as quercetin or butterbur, for additional benefits.

While stinging nettle is generally considered safe for most people, consulting with a healthcare professional before adding it to your daily routine is necessary, especially if you are pregnant, nursing, or taking any medications. Some potential side effects of stinging nettle may include:

- Upset stomach

- Diarrhea

- Sweating

- Skin rash (in rare cases)

Quercetin

Quercetin, a bioflavonoid, can be highly beneficial in managing allergies and asthma. This potent antioxidant is naturally abundant in several fruits and vegetables, including apples, onions, and berries. Its function as a natural antihistamine and anti-inflammatory agent is integral to its ability to alleviate allergy symptoms.

When an allergic reaction occurs, mast cells are stimulated and release histamine, a chemical that triggers allergy symptoms such as sneezing, itching, and congestion. Quercetin also helps stabilize these mast cells, reducing histamine release and alleviating allergy symptoms.

This bioflavonoid is not only helpful for those suffering from seasonal allergies but also offers relief for asthma patients. Asthma, a chronic condition involving inflammation of the airways, can benefit from the anti-inflammatory properties of quercetin. This compound may help soothe inflamed airways, making breathing easier for individuals with asthma.

While quercetin can be obtained naturally from certain foods, it can also be consumed in capsule form as a supplement to ensure adequate and precise intake. The effectiveness of quercetin can be enhanced when combined with certain other substances. Vitamin C and bromelain, an enzyme found in pineapples, are two such substances. Vitamin C can aid in improving the bioavailability of quercetin, while bromelain supports its anti-inflammatory effects.

Anxiety and Stress

Have you ever encountered someone who hasn't experienced stress and anxiety? I'm willing to bet your answer is a resounding "NO!." In fact, anxiety and stress have become all too familiar in our modern world, affecting many individuals and significantly influencing their day-to-day existence. Undeniably, these pervasive issues have become an integral part of our lives, needing our attention and care.

Anxiety is characterized by excessive worry, fear, or nervousness, often disproportionate to the situation. It can manifest in various ways, from generalized anxiety disorder to panic attacks and social anxiety. On the other hand, stress is a natural response to challenging situations or external pressures. While short-term stress can be helpful in certain circumstances, chronic stress can take a toll on our physical and emotional well-being.

The uplifting news is herbal remedies are here to lend a helping hand, providing gentle support in managing anxiety and stress, offering a natural way to promote relaxation, enhance mood, and foster a sense of balance.

While there are numerous herbs with calming and stress-relieving properties, the following four are among the most popular and widely used:

Chamomile

The soothing nature of this herb, scientifically named Matricaria chamomilla, is primarily due to a compound called apigenin. This flavonoid binds to specific receptors in your brain to promote deep relaxation, reduce anxiety, and even facilitate sleep. This makes chamomile a superb ally for those struggling with stress-related sleep disturbances.

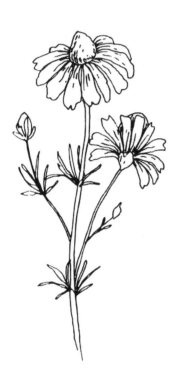

Beyond apigenin, chamomile contains many other chemical compounds contributing to its calming effects. Its unique blend of flavonoids and terpenoids has been found to provide mild sedative effects, making chamomile a natural and gentle way to help calm a racing mind or tense body.

The most common way to harness the calming benefits of chamomile is through a simple herbal tea. Steeping dried chamomile flowers in hot water releases these beneficial compounds, and the very act of sipping warm tea can be a calming ritual. As an herbalist, I often recommend enjoying a cup of chamomile tea as part of a wind-down routine before bed or even during the day when feelings of stress or anxiety start to surface.

Alternatively, chamomile is available in more concentrated forms, such as capsules or tinctures, for those needing a more potent dose. Chamomile essential oil, diluted with a carrier oil, can also be used in aromatherapy or applied topically for a soothing massage, offering yet another pathway for the body to absorb its calming benefits.

Valerian

Valerian root has been used for centuries to treat anxiety, stress, and sleep disorders. It contains compounds interacting with the nervous system to promote relaxation and reduce stress. Valerian (Valeriana officinalis) is usually taken as a supplement in capsule or tincture form, and it's sometimes combined with other calming herbs like passionflower or lemon balm.

Passionflower

Passionflower (Passiflora incarnata) carries a rich legacy of traditional use for its calming and anxiolytic, or anxiety-reducing, properties. Its unique ability to calm the mind and encourage a sense of relaxation is tied to its impact on gamma-aminobutyric acid (GABA). This neurotransmitter helps to quieten neural activity in the brain. By promoting higher GABA levels, passionflower can effectively dial down feelings of anxiety and usher in a sense of calm.

This beautiful vine, renowned for its intricate flowers, provides more than just visual delight. It's a powerful yet gentle herb used for generations to combat restlessness, nervous tension, and sleep disorders. Numerous studies have validated these uses, showing promising results for its application in reducing anxiety and improving sleep quality.

Do you want to know how to enjoy the benefits of this herb? The easiest way is to steep its dried leaves to make a soothing tea; you can also combine it with other calming herbs like chamomile or lemon balm.

Ingredients:

• 1 tablespoon dried chamomile flowers

• 1 tablespoon dried lemon balm leaves

• 1 tablespoon dried passionflower leaves

• 1 teaspoon dried lavender buds

• Honey or natural sweetener (optional)

Instructions:

1. Mix chamomile, lemon balm, passionflower, and lavender in a small bowl.

2. Bring 2 cups of water to a boil, remove from heat, and add two tablespoons of the herbal blend.

3. Cover and let steep for 5-10 minutes. Strain the tea, discarding the spent herbs.

4. Sweeten with honey or preferred sweetener if desired. Enjoy the calming effects.

This recipe makes two servings. Store the leftover dried herbal blend in an airtight container, away from direct sunlight and heat.

If you prefer a more concentrated form, passionflower is also available as a tincture or in capsule form. These can be particularly helpful for managing temporary episodes of anxiety, as they offer a higher concentration of active compounds and are quickly absorbed by the body.

Arthritis and Joint Pain

Arthritis and joint pain are common health issues that can substantially impact a person's mobility, comfort, and overall quality of life. Arthritis is an umbrella term for a group of conditions that cause inflammation and stiffness in the joints, with the two most common types being osteoarthritis and rheumatoid arthritis. Joint pain can also result from various other causes, including injury, overuse, or strain. Successfully managing arthritis and joint pain requires a comprehensive approach that includes making lifestyle changes, engaging in physical therapy, and taking medication to reduce inflammation and improve joint function.

Here are some herbs widely used for their pain-relieving and anti-inflammatory properties:

Ginger

Ginger, the everyday kitchen spice, carries a hidden secret: it's a rich source of potent compounds like gingerols and shogaols. These compounds are the secret agents behind ginger's anti-inflammatory and analgesic properties. So, what does this mean for arthritis and joint pain sufferers? Simply put, ginger may offer a natural solution.

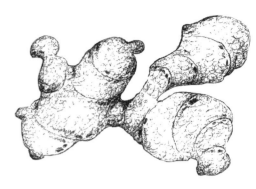

Think of ginger as a super-spy infiltrating your body's inflammatory pathways. Once inside, it doesn't just put up a fight; it actively works to dismantle the chemical processes that cause inflammation and pain. This is especially useful for those struggling with arthritis, a condition characterized by chronic inflammation and joint discomfort.

Now, you might wonder, where can you find this remarkable spice in its natural form? The answer is as fascinating as the spice itself. Ginger is a tropical plant that originated in Southeast Asia. It thrives in rich, moist soil and prefers warm, humid conditions. In the wild, it can be found in countries like India, China, and Nepal. Today, it's also cultivated worldwide in favorable climates, including parts of Africa, the Caribbean, and South America.

But you don't necessarily have to go to the tropics to catch some. Ginger can be readily found in your local supermarket's produce section. It is typically sold in its root form, a thick, knotted rhizome that can be easily peeled and grated. You may also find dried ground ginger in the spice aisle.

To unlock the health-promoting benefits of ginger, consider integrating it into your diet. Grating fresh ginger root into hot water creates a soothing tea while using it to add flavor to your meals brings a delightful twist to your culinary adventures. If the taste is too strong, ginger is also available in more convenient forms, such as capsules, extracts, and even topical creams or balms.

Turmeric

Turmeric, a spice most known for its role in Indian cuisine, offers far more than just a warm, earthy flavor and vibrant color. The active compound in turmeric, called curcumin, boasts substantial anti-inflammatory properties, making turmeric (Curcuma longa) a valuable ally in managing conditions characterized by inflammation, such as arthritis.

Inflammation plays a crucial role in arthritis, leading to the characteristic pain and stiffness experienced by those with the condition. By helping to reduce inflammation, curcumin can consequently help mitigate these symptoms. Several scientific studies have demonstrated turmeric's effectiveness in reducing joint pain and swelling in people with arthritis, often matching the effectiveness of some conventional pain medications but with fewer side effects.

While turmeric can be consumed as a food spice, higher quantities are typically required for therapeutic effects, often achieved through turmeric or curcumin supplements, widely available in capsule form. However, the body does not readily absorb curcumin alone, and it's usually recommended to take it with black pepper or fats to enhance absorption.

Topical use of turmeric is also popular, especially for localized pain and inflammation. Turmeric creams and balms can be applied directly to the affected area, helping to relieve the discomfort.

For a homemade topical application, try this simple turmeric paste: Mix two tablespoons of turmeric powder with enough coconut oil to form a thick paste, then add a generous pinch of black pepper (which contains piperine to enhance absorption). Apply the paste to the painful area and leave it on for about 20 minutes before washing it off. Remember to always do a patch test first to prevent any adverse skin reaction to the paste.

Boswellia

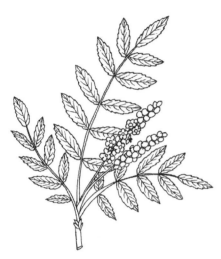

Boswellia, known as Indian frankincense, opens up a world of natural remedies, particularly when treating arthritis and joint pain. With its deeply-rooted Ayurvedic heritage, this plant relieves inflammation-related issues.

Packed with potent anti-inflammatory and analgesic properties, Boswellia works fascinatingly. It targets and suppresses the production of certain compounds within the body that cause inflammation.

The result is a substantial reduction in joint pain and swelling, offering comforting relief to those affected by arthritic conditions.

The appeal of Boswellia isn't solely limited to its benefits but also extends to its accessibility. The plant can be found in many parts of the world, including India and Northern Africa. However, it's important to note that Boswellia is not typically consumed directly from the plant itself. Instead, it is the resin, or sap, obtained from the plant's bark that is utilized for medicinal purposes.

The resin is transformed into a form suitable for human consumption to extract its benefits. This is typically done by turning the resin into a powder, which is then encapsulated or pressed into tablets. The resulting supplement, rich in Boswellia's beneficial compounds, can be easily incorporated into daily routines.

Devil's Claw

Native to southern Africa, devil's Claw (Harpagophytum procumbens) has long been used as a natural remedy for arthritis and joint pain. Its active compounds, harpagosides, have been shown to possess anti-inflammatory and analgesic properties, making it an effective option for those grappling with joint issues. Devil's Claw is typically taken as a supplement in capsule or tablet form or used as a topical cream.

Paul, a retired athlete, struggled with persistent knee pain for years. His symptoms noticeably improved by incorporating turmeric and ginger into his daily routine. The herbal remedies let him embrace his active lifestyle with renewed ease and comfort. Witnessing this transformation reaffirmed my belief in the healing power of herbs.

Colds and Flu

Colds and flu are common viral infections that affect the respiratory system, causing discomfort and symptoms such as sneezing, coughing, sore throat, congestion, and fever. While colds tend to be milder and more short-lived, the flu can be more severe and may even lead to complications in some cases. Different types of viruses cause both colds and flu; although there is no cure for these infections, herbal remedies can help reduce symptoms and shorten recovery time.

The following herbs are among the most widely used for their immune-boosting and symptom-relieving properties:

Echinacea

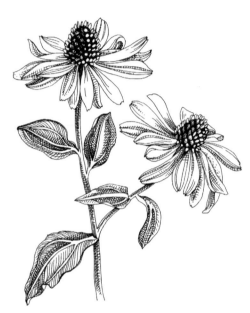

Echinacea, a native North American plant, is prized for its healing properties. It's a holistic superhero known for its anti-inflammatory and antiviral capabilities. Many see it as a natural shield, boosting the body's defense against common ailments like colds and the flu.

The strength of Echinacea stems from the roots, leaves, and flowers of the plant. From these parts, supplements are created that are thought to enhance the immune system and provide respite from respiratory infections. Now, here comes the exciting part: envision a remedy that has the potential to shorten the duration of your illness and alleviate the severity of your symptoms. Enter Echinacea, the enchanting herb with remarkable healing properties.

When you're on the cusp of a cold or flu - when that telltale scratchy throat or runny nose first appears - taking Echinacea can help turn the tide. Studies suggest that if taken at the onset of these symptoms, Echinacea can reduce the duration and intensity of the illness, helping you bounce back faster.

To illustrate the potential benefits of Echinacea more clearly, let's break it down:

- Shorter Illness Duration: Some research indicates that Echinacea may reduce the length of a cold or flu, meaning that you could return to your feet faster, resuming your daily activities with renewed energy.

- Lessened Symptom Severity: Battling a cold or flu can make you miserable. Echinacea may help ease this discomfort by reducing symptoms like a runny nose, sore throat, and fatigue.

- Immune Support: Echinacea is widely known for its immune-boosting properties. Regular use can potentially strengthen your immune system, providing an added layer of protection against seasonal ailments.

Echinacea is available in several forms, such as tea, tincture, capsules, and even throat lozenges. It's like having a natural wellness toolbox at your fingertips! The next time you sense a cold or flu looming, don't forget the potential power of Echinacea.

Elderberry

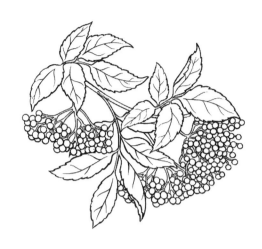

Elderberry, specifically the Sambucus nigra, holds an esteemed place in the arsenal of natural remedies, and for a good reason. This plant's deep, rich berries are brimming with immune-supportive elements and have been used for centuries as a powerful defense against common respiratory ailments like the cold and flu.

One of the standout benefits of elderberry is its rich antioxidant content. These antioxidants shield the body's cells from damage, ultimately supporting overall health and strengthening the immune system. When a cold or the flu is at your doorstep, a body strengthened by elderberries can vigorously fight, possibly helping you ward off the illness before it entirely takes hold.

Moreover, elderberry is recognized for its antiviral properties. It has been observed to hinder the replication of some viruses, potentially reducing the duration of your illness. Imagine the difference between a cold that drags on for a week or more versus one that resolves in a few days. Elderberry might tip the balance in your favor.

Elderberry is commonly consumed as syrup, offering a delightful approach that is often enjoyed by children as well. Here's an essential step-by-step guide on how to make your elderberry syrup at home:

1. Gather your ingredients: About half a cup of dried elderberries, three cups of water, and a cup of raw honey.

2. Combine the elderberries and water in a pot and bring to a boil.

3. Reduce heat and let it simmer for about 45 minutes until the liquid has reduced by half.

4. Strain the mixture into a jar, pressing on the berries to extract as much juice as possible.

5. Once cooled, stir in the honey. Your homemade elderberry syrup is now ready.

Remember, timing is crucial in tapping into elderberry's benefits. As soon as you sense those first inklings of a cold or flu – a tickle in your throat, a slight body ache – that's your signal to grab your trusted elderberry syrup.

Peppermint

Peppermint, scientifically known as Mentha piperita, is a plant often used to treat various health conditions, including the common cold and flu. This versatile herb's potency primarily stems from menthol, a natural compound widely recognized for its therapeutic properties.

One of the most noticeable effects of peppermint in treating cold and flu symptoms is its ability to soothe a sore throat. The cooling sensation of menthol can bring instant relief, helping to reduce the harsh feeling of soreness and irritation that often accompanies these illnesses.

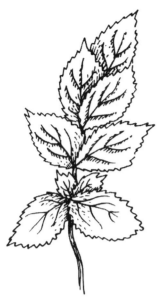

Drinking a hot cup of peppermint tea is a simple and enjoyable way to derive this benefit. You can steep fresh or dried peppermint leaves in boiling water for about ten minutes, strain, and sip slowly. This herbal tea calms your throat and promotes hydration, another key factor aiding your swift return to health.

In addition, peppermint can relieve congestion, a common symptom that can cause significant discomfort when dealing with a cold or flu. The menthol found in peppermint is a helpful ally in thinning mucus and clearing nasal passages, making it easier to breathe and relieve congestion. Its invigorating properties provide a refreshing sensation that promotes a sense of ease and comfort, allowing you to breathe freely once again. Consider adding a few drops of peppermint essential oil to a diffuser or a bowl of hot water and inhale the steam. This form of aromatherapy can provide immediate relief from blocked sinuses and heavy chests.

Lastly, when used as a chest rub, peppermint has the potential to provide relief from persistent coughs. Commercial chest rubs often contain menthol due to its efficacy in calming coughs, but a homemade version can work just as well. You might mix peppermint essential oil with a carrier oil like coconut or almond oil, apply the mixture to your chest, and gently massage it. The warming sensation can help to relax the respiratory muscles and reduce coughing bouts, leading to a more comfortable sleep.

Chapter Two

Digestive and Neurological Issues

Digestive Issues

Digestive issues can encompass a wide range of conditions that affect the gastrointestinal (GI) tract, including heartburn, indigestion, bloating, gas, constipation, and diarrhea. Various factors, such as poor diet, stress, food sensitivities, or an imbalance in the gut microbiome, can cause these issues. While some digestive problems are short-lived and easily manageable, others can become chronic and worsen a person's quality of life.

Here are some herbs widely used for their digestive support properties:

Marshmallow Root

Marshmallow root, scientifically known as Althaea officinalis, is an impressive natural remedy, particularly in addressing digestive ailments such as gastritis, esophagitis, and irritable bowel syndrome (IBS).

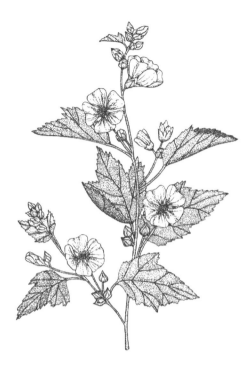

This humble plant is highly regarded for its exceptional soothing and demulcent qualities.

Marshmallow root has a specific property: it is high in mucilage, a type of polysaccharide that becomes slippery and gel-like when wet. Because of its function, it can form a protective coating in the gastrointestinal tract. As a result, it functions as a barrier against inflammation and irritation, easing the delicate tissues of the digestive system.

Individuals dealing with digestive conditions can utilize marshmallow root in various forms to tap into its healing potential. For tea lovers, marshmallow root can be steeped in hot water to create a relaxing beverage. Tinctures, another form, offer a liquid solution that can be taken directly or mixed into water or juice. Alternatively, marshmallow root is available in capsule form for those who prefer a more concentrated form, providing an easy and convenient option.

Regarding sourcing marshmallow root, the plant is native to Europe, Western Asia, and North Africa. However, it has been successfully cultivated in other parts of the world, including North America. The roots are harvested in late autumn or early spring for medicinal use.

For those curious about growing their marshmallow plants, it's worth noting that they are perennial, meaning they come back year after year. These plants thrive in sunny locations and prefer moist, well-drained soils for optimal growth.

Fennel

Fennel (Foeniculum vulgare) is a versatile and aromatic herb valued for its potential benefits in traditional medicine, particularly for addressing digestive discomforts. With its rich essential oils, vitamins, and minerals, fennel offers a range of properties that can help alleviate gastrointestinal issues.

Fennel is believed to possess antispasmodic, carminative, and anti-inflammatory properties, which can aid in addressing several digestive concerns:

- Reducing Bloating and Gas: Fennel's carminative properties help expel gas from the digestive system, relieving bloating and abdominal discomfort.

- Alleviating Abdominal Pain: The antispasmodic properties of fennel can help relax the muscles in the gastrointestinal tract, easing cramps and reducing pain.

- Promoting Healthy Digestion: Fennel stimulates the production of digestive enzymes, which can improve the breakdown and absorption of nutrients from food.

- Regulating Bowel Movements: By supporting healthy digestion and relaxing the intestinal muscles, fennel can help control bowel movements and prevent constipation.

There are several methods to infuse fennel into your daily routine to reap its digestive benefits:

1. Tea: Fennel tea can be prepared by steeping crushed fennel seeds or fresh leaves in hot water. To make fennel tea, add 1-2 teaspoons of crushed fennel seeds or fresh leaves to a cup of boiling water, let it steep for about 10 minutes, then strain and enjoy.

2. Chewing Seeds: Fennel seeds can be chewed directly after meals to aid digestion and freshen breathing. Consume a small spoonful of seeds and chew them slowly to release their beneficial oils.

3. Supplements: Fennel is available in various supplement forms, such as capsules or extracts. Follow the recommended dosage on the product label and consult a healthcare professional before taking any supplement.

Fennel is a perennial herb that grows naturally in various parts of the world, including the Mediterranean region, Western Asia, and Europe. It is often cultivated in gardens and can be produced from seeds or transplants. Fennel can be found in the wild, along roadsides, and in open fields, but it is crucial to ensure proper identification before harvesting from a natural environment.

Cumin

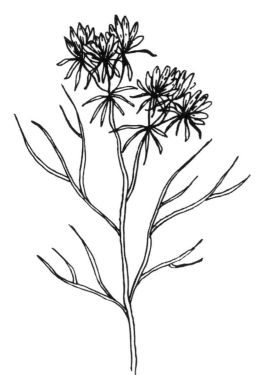

Cumin, a spice derived from the plant Cuminum cyminum, has been a beloved ingredient in many culinary traditions across the world. The spice, which offers a distinctive, earthy flavor, is not only celebrated for its culinary use but also for its potential health benefits. In the ancient medical systems of Ayurveda and Traditional Chinese Medicine, cumin has long been valued as a powerful herbal remedy.

General Health Uses

Respiratory Health: Cumin has been traditionally used to address respiratory conditions, thanks to its anti-inflammatory and anti-microbial properties.

Diabetes Management: Some research suggests cumin may play a role in managing blood sugar levels, making it a potential support for people with diabetes.

Iron Deficiency Anemia: As a good source of iron, cumin may help in combating iron deficiency anemia.

While these uses are important, it is cumin's role in promoting digestive health that truly sets it apart.

A Digestive Powerhouse

Cumin has long been a trusted ally for maintaining digestive health. It is frequently used to manage various digestive disorders due to its carminative, stimulant, and anti-spasmodic properties.

- Aiding Digestion – Cumin is believed to stimulate the secretion of pancreatic enzymes, which are necessary for proper digestion and nutrient assimilation. This stimulation can help to enhance overall digestion, making it easier for the body to process foods and absorb nutrients.

- Relieving Gas and Bloating – As a carminative, cumin can help to relieve symptoms of gas and bloating. By promoting the expulsion of gas from the body, cumin can help to alleviate discomfort and prevent excessive gas accumulation.

- Alleviating IBS Symptoms – Cumin may also help to alleviate symptoms of Irritable Bowel Syndrome (IBS). Its anti-spasmodic properties can help to reduce abdominal pain and cramping often associated with this condition.

- Combating Indigestion – Traditionally, cumin has been used to treat indigestion. It is often taken in the form of tea - simply steep cumin seeds in hot water, strain, and drink. This warm cumin tea can help to stimulate digestion and soothe the stomach.

Slippery Elm

Slippery Elm (Ulmus rubra) is a valuable herb for alleviating digestive issues, including heartburn, acid reflux, gastritis, and inflammatory bowel conditions such as ulcerative colitis and Crohn's disease. Traditionally used to calm and protect the lining of the digestive tract, Slippery Elm derives its efficacy from its high mucilage content, which forms a gel-like substance when combined with water. This gel creates a protective barrier against irritation and inflammation in the gastrointestinal tract.

The properties of Slippery Elm can help address several digestive concerns:

- Heartburn and Acid Reflux: Slippery Elm's mucilage content coats the esophagus, relieving the burning sensation caused by stomach acid.

- Gastritis: The protective barrier formed by Slippery Elm's mucilage can help shield the stomach lining from irritation and inflammation, promoting healing in cases of gastritis.

- Inflammatory Bowel Conditions: Slippery Elm may help reduce inflammation and irritation in the digestive tract, relieving individuals with ulcerative colitis or Crohn's disease.

There are several methods to incorporate Slippery Elm into your daily routine to reap its digestive benefits:

1. Tea: Prepare Slippery Elm tea by steeping 1-2 teaspoons of the powdered bark in hot water for about 5 minutes. Strain and enjoy as needed.

2. Capsules: Slippery Elm is available in capsule form, offering a convenient way to consume the herb. Follow the recommended dosage on the product label and consult a healthcare professional before using any supplement.

3. Powder: Mix Slippery Elm powder with water to create a soothing drink, or add it to smoothies for added benefits. Start with a small amount, such as 1 teaspoon, and gradually increase the dosage as needed.

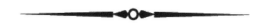

Among the herbs we've previously explored, peppermint and ginger are known to relieve stomach and intestinal issues. The menthol in peppermint relaxes the GI tract's smooth muscles, reducing spasms, cramping, and easing indigestion and IBS symptoms. Ginger has carminative and anti-inflammatory properties, helping to reduce gas, bloating, cramping, nausea, and indigestion.

Headaches and Migraines

Headaches and migraines are common ailments that affect millions of people worldwide. While headaches can be caused by various factors such as tension, dehydration, or sinus issues, migraines are a more severe form of headache, often accompanied by nausea, sensitivity to light and sound, and visual disturbances.

Many people seek natural alternatives to manage these debilitating conditions, and herbal remedies can offer practical solutions to alleviate symptoms.

Here are some of the most common herbal remedies for headaches and migraines:

Feverfew

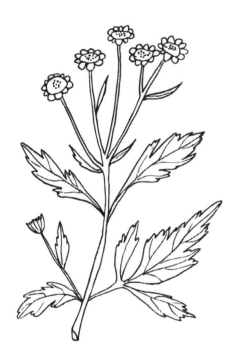

Feverfew, scientifically known as Tanacetum parthenium, opens up new possibilities for individuals dealing with recurrent headaches, especially migraines. A sturdy, aromatic herb with daisy-like flowers, feverfew is far from being an ordinary garden resident. Its medicinal prowess has been revered since ancient times, earning it a respected position in the world of natural remedies.

As we delve into the essence of this remarkable plant, we uncover parthenolide, the primary active compound that steals the spotlight. This exceptional ingredient acts as a skilled artisan, meticulously crafting an internal environment that is less susceptible to migraines. It achieves this by addressing two main factors responsible for these debilitating headaches: inflammation and constriction of blood vessels. With its precise actions, parthenolide aims to bring relief and establish a sanctuary within the body, reducing the likelihood of migraines taking hold.

Imagine the body as a peaceful city. Inflammation is like a sudden, disruptive protest, causing chaos and discomfort. Like an adept peacekeeper, Parthenolide steps in, effectively calming the turmoil, reducing inflammation, and restoring order within the body's intricate biological network.

Meanwhile, blood vessels in the brain can sometimes behave like rush hour traffic, tightening and constricting, leading to a painful gridlock – the migraine. Parthenolide again takes charge, acting like a proficient traffic controller, maintaining a smooth flow by preventing this constriction.

Yet, the wonders of feverfew do not stop at parthenolide alone. The herb is a reservoir of other beneficial compounds, such as flavonoids and sesquiterpene lactones, all contributing to its remarkable healing properties.

Butterbur

Butterbur (Petasites hybridus) is a herb with a long history of use in traditional medicine.

The primary benefits of butterbur stem from its unique properties, which are especially helpful for those who suffer from headaches and migraines. These benefits include:

- Anti-inflammatory Effects: Butterbur contains compounds that can help reduce inflammation in the body, which may contribute to headache and migraine relief. By minimizing inflammation, butterbur can potentially alleviate pain and discomfort associated with these conditions.

- Antispasmodic Action: The antispasmodic properties of butterbur can help relax the muscles and blood vessels in the head, which may be particularly beneficial for those experiencing tension headaches or migraines. By easing muscle tension and promoting blood flow, butterbur can provide relief from headache-related symptoms.

If you are interested in trying Butterbur as a natural remedy, the following steps can help ensure proper usage:

1. Choose the Right Form: Butterbur is available in various forms, including capsules, tablets, and tinctures. For beginners, capsules or tablets are often the most convenient and accessible options.

2. Follow the Recommended Dosage: Always adhere to the recommended dosage instructions on the product label, as the appropriate dosage may vary depending on the specific product and formulation.

3. Consult a Healthcare Professional: Before incorporating butterbur into your daily routine, it is better to consult with a healthcare professional, especially if you are pregnant, nursing, or taking any medications.

Lavender

While lavender (Lavandula angustifolia) originated in the Mediterranean region, its cultivation has extended worldwide. Today, lavender can be found in various corners of the globe, from Europe to Africa and Asia. Lavender plants can be grown in gardens, and their flowers can be harvested to extract the essential oil.

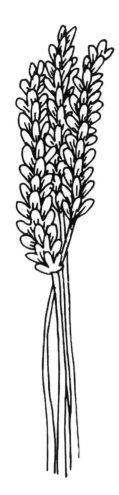

Lavender essential oil possesses a range of properties that can aid in relieving pain and alleviating the stress often associated with headaches and migraines:

Pain Relief: Lavender essential oil contains analgesic properties that can ease pain, including that of headaches and migraines.

Relaxation: The calming scent of lavender essential oil promotes relaxation, helping to relieve tension that can contribute to headaches and migraines.

Stress Reduction: Lavender essential oil has been shown to have a soothing effect on the nervous system, which can help reduce stress and anxiety that may trigger migraines. There are several methods to integrate lavender essential oil into your routine to get its headache and migraine-relieving benefits:

Inhalation: Add a few drops of lavender essential oil to a diffuser or a bowl of hot water, and inhale the aromatic steam to help reduce headache and migraine severity.

Topical Application: Dilute lavender essential oil with a carrier oil (such as coconut or almond oil) and gently massage it onto the temples, forehead, and neck to alleviate headache pain.

Aromatherapy: Use lavender essential oil in an aromatherapy bath, adding a few drops to warm bathwater to promote relaxation and relieve headache symptoms.

When it comes to lavender essential oil, choosing wisely is key. Don't settle for anything less than a high-quality, pure product from a trusted supplier. Opting for synthetic or adulterated oils may not provide the same benefits that you're seeking. You can find lavender essential oil in health food stores, specialty shops, and online retailers.

I recommend trying this soothing herbal tea blend when you have a headache. Combine one teaspoon of dried feverfew leaves, one teaspoon of dried lavender flowers, and one teaspoon of dried peppermint leaves in a teapot or large mug. Pour boiling water over the herbs, cover, and steep for 10-15 minutes. Strain the tea and enjoy it when symptoms arise or as a preventive measure.

Chapter Three

Gender-Specific and Skin Conditions

Skin Conditions

We've all experienced it at some point in our lives—those common yet troublesome skin conditions that can disrupt our peace of mind. Whether it's acne, eczema, psoriasis, or dermatitis, these dermatological challenges bring along unwelcome symptoms like itching, redness, dryness, and inflammation.

The good news is that there are natural remedies and strategies to help address and manage these common skin concerns. Many people prefer natural alternatives to traditional therapies for their skin issues and overall skin health. With a holistic approach and the power of nature, we can find effective and practical solutions that promote healthy skin and boost confidence. Let's explore these options together and unlock the secrets to radiant skin.

Here are some of the most common herbal solutions to calm and nourish the skin:

Aloe Vera

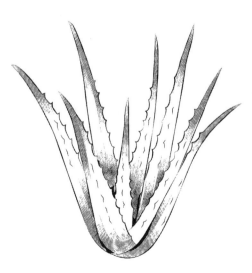

Originating from the Arabian Peninsula, this plant (scientifically known as Aloe barbadensis), with its spiky leaves and hardy disposition, is now found worldwide. Within the thick, aloe-filled leaves lies a powerhouse of nutrients and beneficial compounds that make it an exceptional choice for addressing numerous skin conditions.

Whether it's soothing burns, calming sunburns, alleviating insect bites, relieving rashes, or healing other skin irritations, aloe vera's applications are impressively broad. The efficacy of aloe vera for these conditions can be attributed to the gel extracted from the plant's leaves, which is packed with an array of vitamins, minerals, enzymes, and amino acids.

The primary reason behind aloe vera's ability to revitalize and repair skin is its potent moisturizing, anti-inflammatory, and antimicrobial properties. The gel naturally hydrates the skin, making it an ideal choice for dry skin conditions. Simultaneously, it can reduce redness and inflammation associated with various skin irritations, promoting the healing of damaged skin tissue.

What sets aloe vera apart is its ability to stimulate collagen production, a protein crucial for skin strength and elasticity. With increased collagen, the skin becomes more supple and resilient, reducing the appearance of wrinkles and fine lines. This has made aloe vera a sought-after ingredient in anti-aging skincare products.

Applying aloe vera directly to the skin is simple. One can cut a leaf from the plant, slice it open, and scoop out the healing gel concealed within. Apply this gel to the affected area and let it absorb into the skin for the best results.

For those without access to a fresh aloe plant, there's no need to fret. A wide range of commercially made aloe vera gels or lotions are readily available in health food stores and pharmacies. However, it's important to select a product that contains a high percentage of aloe vera and has minimal additional ingredients to ensure effectiveness.

Calendula

Due to its anti-inflammatory and antibacterial features, Calendula (Calendula officinalis) is commonly used to relieve and heal various skin conditions, including cuts, burns, and rashes. It can be applied on the skin as an infused oil, cream, or salve.

Tea Tree

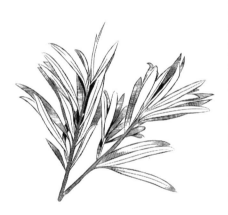

Native to Australia, tea tree oil is extracted from the Melaleuca alternifolia plant leaves and is traditionally used for its healing properties. As a potent antimicrobial and anti-inflammatory agent, tea tree oil is highly effective in treating numerous skin conditions, including acne, athlete's foot, nail fungus, and other bacterial or fungal skin infections.

Say goodbye to acne-causing bacteria and inflammation with the powerful compounds found in tea tree oil. Its magic lies in terpinene-4-ol, which fights breakouts and reduces their severity. But that's not all! Tea tree oil's anti-inflammatory properties also work wonders for soothing eczema, psoriasis, and dermatitis. Embrace the natural goodness of tea tree oil and experience its transformative effects on your skin.

However, remember that when using tea tree oil topically, it's necessary to dilute it with a carrier oil, such as almond, jojoba, or coconut oil, to prevent skin irritation. A typical dilution ratio is 2-5% tea tree oil, translating to 12-30 drops per ounce of carrier oil. You can also find tea tree oil in various skincare products, such as cleansers, toners, and spot treatments, specifically formulated for safe and effective use.

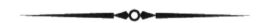

A simple recipe for a soothing skin salve involves combining Calendula and chamomile. First, create an infused oil by placing 1/2 cup of dried calendula flowers and 1/2 cup of dried chamomile flowers in a jar. Cover the herbs with a carrier oil, such as almond or olive oil, and let them steep in a warm, dark place for 2-4 weeks. Strain the oil and combine it with 1/4 cup of beeswax, melting the mixture in a double boiler. Pour the liquid into tins or jars and let it cool before using it on irritated or inflamed skin.

Sleep Disorders

Insomnia, sleep apnea, restless leg syndrome, and narcolepsy can lead to chronic sleep deprivation, resulting in a weakened immune system, impaired cognitive function, and increased risk of chronic diseases.

Nowadays, many individuals seek natural solutions to enhance their sleep quality without worrying about dependence or unwanted side effects. So, let's explore the realm of natural sleep remedies and uncover some of the most common and trusted options to help you achieve that well-deserved restful slumber.

Valerian

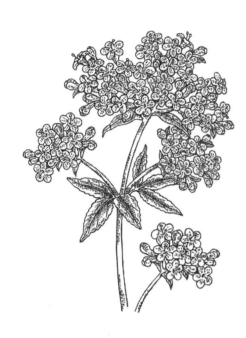

Valerian, a perennial plant with roots in Europe and Asia, carries a rich history of medicinal use. Its intriguing legacy can be traced back to the time of ancient Greece and Rome, where it was highly regarded for its healing properties.

The calming effects of valerian are attributed to the synergy of various compounds found within the plant. Among them, valerenic acid, isovaleric acid, and several alkaloids are thought to be particularly influential. These compounds work within the intricate systems of the brain, mainly by boosting the availability of a crucial neurotransmitter called gamma-aminobutyric acid (GABA). The role of GABA is to regulate nerve impulses, and its enhanced presence in the brain brings about a state of relaxation.

There are several forms to consider to experience the beneficial effects of valerian. Tinctures and capsules offer concentrated dosages, but there's a certain charm in the simplicity and ritual of brewing valerian tea. Preparing valerian tea involves a teaspoon of dried valerian root and a cup of boiling water. Allowing this mixture to steep for 5-10 minutes extracts the beneficial compounds from the root. After straining the tea, it's ready to be enjoyed. Consuming this calming infusion about 30 minutes before bedtime can help set the stage for a restful night's sleep.

Apart from the traditional methods, valerian root is also used in essential oils for aromatherapy, which is another way to enjoy its calming benefits. The aroma of valerian oil can be inhaled directly or diffused in the bedroom to provide a tranquil sleep environment.

California Poppy

California poppy (Eschscholzia californica) is a gentle sedative herb known for its ability to alleviate anxiety and promote restful sleep.

The calming properties of California poppy can help address various sleep-related issues:

Anxiety Relief - California poppy has anxiolytic effects, which can help reduce anxiety levels and create a more relaxed state conducive to sleep.

Sleep Promotion - The herb's sedative properties can encourage restful sleep by calming the nervous system and promoting relaxation.

Mild Side Effects - Unlike stronger sedatives, California poppy is generally well-tolerated and does not typically cause grogginess or other undesirable side effects.

You can infuse it into your routine as tea, tincture, or capsules to enjoy its benefits. Always follow recommended dosages and consult a healthcare professional before using any supplement.

Here are some curious facts about California Poppy:

- State Flower: California poppy is the official state flower of California and is celebrated annually on California Poppy Day (April 6).

- Vibrant Colors: The plant is known for its bright orange flowers, which can also be found in shades of yellow, pink, and red.

- Drought Tolerance: California poppy is a drought-tolerant plant, making it an excellent option for water-wise gardens in arid regions.

- Pollinator Attraction: The colorful flowers of the California poppy attract a variety of pollinators, including bees and butterflies.

Lemon Balm

Lemon balm, a fragrant herb from the mint family, offers an intriguing foray into natural remedies, especially concerning sleep disorders. With a history steeped in centuries of use, this remarkable plant has emerged as a superstar among natural remedies, particularly concerning sleep disorders. Known for its incredible ability to calm the nervous system, lemon balm has become a trusted ally for those seeking respite from stress, relief from anxiety, and the sweet embrace of restful sleep.

The relaxing properties of lemon balm are attributed to its unique composition. Two primary active compounds, rosmarinic acid and various terpenes, play vital roles in engendering its soothing effects. These compounds interact with our brain chemistry, particularly by enhancing the availability of a neurotransmitter called gamma-aminobutyric acid (GABA). This vital neurotransmitter is instrumental in regulating nerve impulses, leading to a state of relaxation when its levels are increased. It's interesting to note that this mechanism shares similarities with valerian.

Harnessing the benefits of lemon balm is a relatively straightforward process, even for beginners. The herb can be consumed as a relaxing tea or taken in capsule form for convenience. To prepare the tea, you need a teaspoon of dried leaves to craft a cup of lemon balm tea. Add this to a cup of boiling water and let the mixture steep for 5-10 minutes. Once the tea is strained, it's ready for consumption. Imbibing this aromatic infusion about 30 minutes before bedtime can help set the stage for a peaceful night's sleep.

Lemon balm can be enjoyed in different forms. You can use its fresh or dried leaves to add a lemony flavor to your cooking. Additionally, lemon balm is available as a tincture or essential oil, which can be applied topically or diffused for its calming scent.

Dill

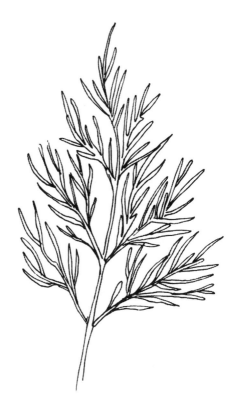

Dill, scientifically known as Anethum graveolens, is a popular herb recognized by its soft, feathery leaves and distinct aroma. Predominantly used as a flavor-enhancing ingredient in cooking, it is also renowned for its variety of medicinal properties that have been utilized across different cultures for centuries.

Here's a brief overview of some of dill's common uses before we delve into its role in managing sleep disorders:

Digestive Health: Dill is often used in traditional medicine as a remedy for digestive issues, helping to alleviate symptoms such as gas, bloating, and stomach discomfort.

Menstrual Cramps: The antispasmodic properties of dill can help ease menstrual cramps and discomfort.

Respiratory Health: Traditionally, dill has been used to relieve coughs and cold symptoms, owing to its antibacterial and antiviral properties.

<u>Dill and Sleep Disorders</u>

Dill is rich in flavonoids and B-complex vitamins, both of which have been shown to stimulate the secretion of certain enzymes that have calming and hypnotic effects. This, in turn, can contribute to better sleep quality. Dill's essential oil is particularly noteworthy for its high concentration of these beneficial compounds.

Many people suffering from insomnia or other sleep disorders turn to a cup of warm dill tea before bed. The soothing, slightly tangy flavor and aroma of the tea can aid in relaxation, while the aforementioned properties get to work on promoting a restful slumber.

Furthermore, the aroma of dill essential oil, when used in aromatherapy, can also help create a calming atmosphere conducive to sleep. Diffusing a few drops of the oil in your bedroom before you retire for the night may help ease you into a deeper, more peaceful sleep.

As always, while dill is generally safe for consumption in culinary amounts, it's prudent to consult with a healthcare provider before using it or any other herb as a therapeutic remedy, especially for persistent sleep disorders.

If you are looking for a recipe to create a relaxing bedtime tea blend, I suggest combining equal parts of dried valerian, chamomile, passionflower, and lemon balm. To make the tea, add one teaspoon of the blended herbs to a cup of boiling water and let it steep for 5-10 minutes. Strain the tea and enjoy it about 30 minutes before bedtime to encourage restful sleep.

Women's Health Issues

Women's health issues comprehend a wide range of conditions unique to or more prevalent in women, such as menstrual discomfort, hormonal imbalances, menopause symptoms, and reproductive health concerns. Here are some herbal remedies to address these issues:

Black Cohosh

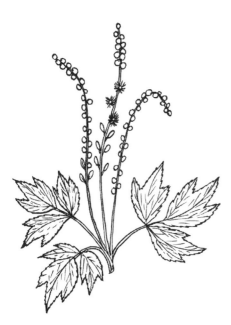

Black Cohosh (Actaea racemosa) holds a rich history deeply rooted in traditional healing practices. Native American healers have long revered this powerful herb for its diverse therapeutic properties. It was highly regarded for its remarkable efficacy in alleviating various conditions and fostering overall health and vitality. As European settlers arrived, they also recognized the value of Black Cohosh and incorporated it into their healing practices. This esteemed herb continues to be utilized for its potential health benefits, making it a valuable addition to natural remedies.

The various properties of Black Cohosh make it an effective natural remedy for:

Menopause Symptom Relief - Black Cohosh's active compounds, such as triterpene glycosides and isoflavones, exhibit estrogen-like effects that help restore hormonal balance, relieving symptoms like hot flashes, night sweats, mood swings, and sleep disturbances.

Premenstrual Syndrome (PMS) Management - The herb has been used to tackle PMS symptoms, including cramps, bloating, irritability, and mood changes. Its anti-inflammatory and antispasmodic properties can help relieve pain and discomfort.

Hormonal Balance Support - Black Cohosh may help regulate hormonal fluctuations, promoting overall reproductive health and well-being.

Black Cohosh can be consumed as a tea, prepared by steeping 1-2 teaspoons of dried root in hot water for around 10 minutes. It is also available as a tincture, providing a convenient usage method. Additionally, those who seek standardized dosages might opt for capsules. In all cases, it's recommended to adhere to the dosage guidelines provided on the product label and consult a healthcare professional before use.

Raspberry Leaf

Raspberry leaf, scientifically known as Rubus idaeus, boasts a treasure trove of vitamins, minerals, and antioxidants, transforming it into a nutritional powerhouse that nourishes the body from within.

Did you know that the raspberry leaf has beneficial effects on the uterus? In fact, it is believed to tone and strengthen uterine muscles, an action that can reduce menstrual cramping and foster more regular, balanced menstrual cycles. Women who have incorporated raspberry leaf into their routines often report noticeable improvements, endorsing its beneficial impact.

Let's explore the delightful ways to savor the goodness of raspberry leaf. Tea tops the list, offering a simple and enjoyable method of consumption. Imagine preparing a steaming cup of raspberry leaf tea, steeping one to two teaspoons of dried leaves in boiling water for 10-15 minutes. After straining, you're left with a warm, soothing beverage that you can savor once or twice daily, all while reaping potential health benefits.

There are other options for those who might not be keen on tea. Raspberry leaf is also available in capsule and tincture forms, providing convenient alternatives that fit easily into any routine.

You might be thinking, where can I find raspberry leaf? Raspberry plants actually grow widely in the wild and are cultivated in many parts of the world. While they're known for their tasty berries, the leaves can be harvested for medicinal use. You can find dried raspberry leaves in health food stores, online, or you might even consider growing your raspberry plants. Cultivating your own plants gives you a fresh, readily available supply of leaves and the added benefit of delicious raspberries.

Majoran

Marjoram, a well-known culinary herb, has long held a cherished place in traditional healing practices. Also known as sweet marjoram or Origanum majorana, this perennial plant belongs to the mint family and is native to the Mediterranean region. Beyond the kitchen, it has been widely used in folk medicine to help address a variety of health conditions. But of all the possible applications, its benefits for women's health stand out as especially noteworthy.

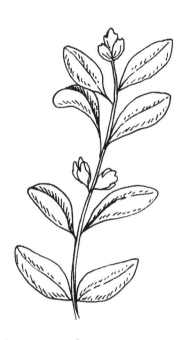

Alleviating Menstrual Discomfort

One of the most common uses of marjoram in women's health is the alleviation of menstrual discomfort. For many women, menstruation is accompanied by painful cramps, often referred to as dysmenorrhea. Marjoram, with its antispasmodic properties, has been used to soothe these muscle contractions and relieve cramping.

A common way to utilize marjoram for menstrual pain is through a warm infusion or tea. A few teaspoons of dried marjoram steeped in hot water can make a soothing drink, believed to help ease the discomfort. Additionally, the essential oil of marjoram can be used in a warm compress or diluted for a gentle abdominal massage.

Menopause Support

As women transition into menopause, they often experience a wide range of symptoms, including hot flashes, mood swings, sleep disturbances, and night sweats. Some research suggests that marjoram may help manage these menopause-related symptoms.

The herb is often used in aromatherapy to manage mood swings and anxiety related to menopause. The essential oil, when used in a diffuser or added to a warm bath, may provide a calming and balancing effect.

Furthermore, marjoram is a source of phytoestrogens, plant compounds that can act similarly to the hormone estrogen in the body. While more research is needed to understand the potential role of phytoestrogens in menopause symptom management, some women find them helpful.

Promoting Hormonal Balance

Interestingly, marjoram has also been traditionally used to help balance hormones in women. Some preliminary studies suggest that regular consumption of marjoram tea may have a beneficial effect on hormonal profile and insulin sensitivity in women with Polycystic Ovary Syndrome (PCOS).

Though the research in this area is not definitive, it provides an intriguing basis for further studies on marjoram's potential role in hormonal health.

In conclusion, while marjoram is best known as a flavorful addition to our meals, its use extends far beyond the culinary world. For centuries, it has been used to address a variety of women's health issues, reflecting its significant role in traditional herbal medicine. However, as always, it's important to consult with a healthcare professional before incorporating herbal remedies into your routine. More research is needed to fully understand marjoram's therapeutic potential and safety.

Vitex

Also known as chasteberry, this small shrub produces fruits that contain compounds believed to influence the pituitary gland, helping regulate the production of hormones such as estrogen and progesterone. As a result, vitex has been effective in easing premenstrual syndrome (PMS) symptoms, including mood swings, breast tenderness, and bloating. Additionally, it has been used to alleviate menopause-related symptoms like hot flashes, mood changes, and sleep disturbances.

Vitex (Vitex agnus-castus) is a popular choice for women with irregular menstrual cycles, as it aids in establishing a more regular cycle. Furthermore, it has been utilized to support fertility by regulating hormone levels in women who face challenges in conceiving. Vitex is available in various forms, including tinctures, capsules, and teas, allowing for convenient intake according to individual preferences.

Dong Quai

Dong Quai (Angelica sinensis) is a traditional Chinese herb suitable for balancing hormones and supporting women's reproductive health.

The various properties of Dong Quai make it a valuable natural remedy for addressing women's health concerns:

- Hormone Balance: Dong Quai is believed to help balance estrogen levels, contributing to a more regular menstrual cycle and reducing menopausal symptoms.

- Menstrual Discomfort Relief: The herb's antispasmodic and anti-inflammatory properties can help alleviate cramps, bloating, and other menstrual discomforts.

- Menopausal Symptom Relief: Dong Quai can help relieve common menopausal symptoms, such as hot flashes, night sweats, and mood swings.

There are several methods to integrate Dong Quai into your routine:

1. Tea: Prepare Dong Quai tea by steeping 1-2 teaspoons of the dried root in hot water for about 10 minutes. Strain and enjoy as needed.

2. Tincture: Dong Quai is available in tincture form, offering a convenient way to consume the herb. Follow the recommended dosage on the product label and consult a healthcare professional before using any supplement.

3. Capsules: You can consume Dong Quai in capsule form if you prefer a more standardized dosage. Follow the product label's recommended dosage and consult a healthcare professional before using any supplement.

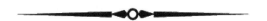

Tea blend recipe - Combine equal parts of dried vitex, black cohosh, raspberry leaf, and dong quai. To make the tea, add one teaspoon of the blended herbs to a cup of boiling water and let it steep for 10-15 minutes. Strain the tea and enjoy it once or twice a day to help support women's well-being.

Men's Health Issues

Hormonal imbalances, prostate health, erectile dysfunction, and reproductive concerns are all examples of men's health problems. Men can care for their health and improve their general quality of life by incorporating natural remedies into a balanced lifestyle. Here we will review some of the most prevalent herbal remedies for men's medical issues and a simple recipe to get you started.

Saw Palmetto

Originating from the southeastern United States, Saw palmetto (Serenoa repens) produces berries that pack a powerful punch. From supporting prostate health to potentially combating hair loss, saw palmetto berries have an array of applications deeply rooted in traditional herbal medicine.

The saw palmetto berries are sources of fatty acids and phytosterols, compounds that have been shown to reduce inflammation and inhibit the conversion of testosterone into dihydrotestosterone (DHT). DHT is a hormone that, when in abundance, can cause complications like benign prostatic hyperplasia (BPH), a common condition affecting older men where the prostate gland becomes enlarged, leading to difficulties with urination. High levels of DHT are also associated with male pattern baldness, making saw palmetto a potential natural remedy for hair loss.

Saw palmetto supplements are widely available and often recommended for their ease of use and standardized dosages. Saw palmetto can also be consumed as a tea, though its taste is somewhat bitter.

To prepare saw palmetto tea, steep the berries in hot water for about 15 minutes, strain, and then drink. You can add honey or another sweetener to make the taste more palatable.

Panax Ginseng

Panax ginseng, also referred to as Korean or Asian ginseng, proves to be a valuable companion for individuals grappling with fatigue or seeking a natural energy boost. But the benefits don't stop there.

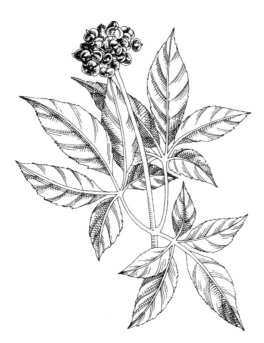

Panax ginseng is also believed to be a potent stress reducer, helping to create a sense of calm and balance amidst the hustle and bustle of modern life.

When it comes to sexual health, Panax ginseng steps up once again. It enhances sexual function and libido, fostering improved well-being and intimacy. Studies suggest that it may help alleviate erectile dysfunction and promote healthy testosterone levels, leading to enhanced sexual desire and performance.

So, how can you incorporate Panax ginseng into your routine? The root of the Panax ginseng plant is typically consumed in one of several forms: fresh, dried (also known as white ginseng), or steamed and dried (also known as red ginseng). Each form is available as a tea, extract, powder, or capsule, allowing you to choose the option that best fits your lifestyle and preferences.

As for sourcing Panax ginseng, it is cultivated primarily in Korea, China, and other parts of East Asia. You can find Panax ginseng products in health food stores, pharmacies, and online.

Maca

Maca, scientifically known as Lepidium meyenii, grows in Peru's harsh climates of the Andes mountains. This root vegetable, part of the crucifer family, has been heralded for its adaptogenic properties for thousands of years. Maca, a nutrient-dense root, is renowned for its rich composition of vitamins, minerals, and amino acids. Indigenous communities have long valued maca for its ability to enhance energy, stamina, and fertility.

It is believed to work on the endocrine system to help balance the production of hormones in both men and women. For men, this balance is crucial for many aspects of health, including mood, growth, sexual development, and libido.

Further, Maca has been cited in numerous studies for its positive effects on male fertility. Specifically, it has been observed to support sperm production and motility, vital factors for male fertility. This is particularly important today, where many environmental factors can negatively affect these parameters.

Maca's rich, nutty flavor lends itself well to various dishes, making it a versatile addition to your diet. For instance, Maca powder can be easily incorporated into your meals. You might add a spoonful to your morning smoothie or oatmeal, sprinkle it over yogurt or cereal, or even blend it into soups or stews. The key is to start with a small amount and gradually increase, as its robust flavor can be overpowering.

Apart from the powder form, Maca is also available in capsules and tinctures, providing a more concentrated dose that can be easily incorporated into your daily routine.

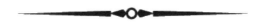

Maca Energy Smoothie

Ingredients:

- 1 cup unsweetened almond milk
- 1 banana
- 1 tablespoon almond butter
- 1 tablespoon chia seeds
- 1 teaspoon maca powder
- 1/2 teaspoon cinnamon
- A handful of ice cubes

Instructions:

1. Combine all ingredients in a blender and blend until smooth and creamy.

2. Pour into a glass and enjoy immediately.

BOOK III

HERBAL REMEDIES FOR CHRONIC CONDITIONS

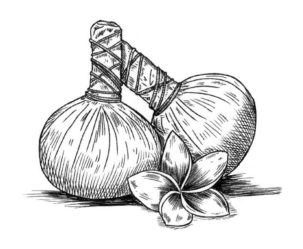

AMBER WHITMORE

Introduction

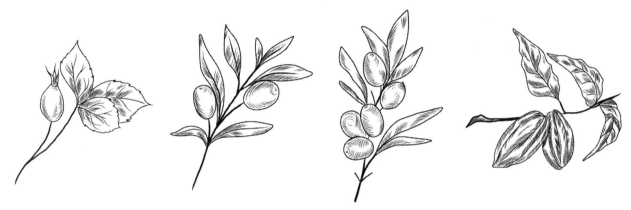

As a herbalist, I've witnessed firsthand the extraordinary power of herbal medicines in improving the lives of individuals with chronic health conditions. Herbs can remarkably support the body's healing processes and foster long-term well-being, benefiting areas such as cardiovascular health and cognitive function.

For instance, I've had clients with high blood pressure who have incorporated hawthorn into their daily routines, effectively controlling their blood pressure levels. Similarly, I've seen the transformative effects of herbs like turmeric, which have alleviated inflammation and relieved pain in individuals with chronic joint disorders. These personal experiences highlight the incredible potential of herbs to positively transform lives and promote optimal health.

Please bear in mind that herbal medicines should be taken alongside, not in place of, conventional medical care. Before adopting herbal remedies into your treatment plan, you must consult with your healthcare professional because they can interact with pharmaceuticals and affect individual health issues differently.

Get ready to explore together the herbal medicines that have been shown to benefit cardiovascular health, aid in diabetes control, support immunological function, promote liver and kidney health, enhance memory and cognitive function, and improve respiratory health. We will discuss the specific herbs that are known for their usefulness in each area, as well as provide practical strategies for incorporating these potent plant allies into your daily routine.

Chapter One
Systemic Chronic Conditions

Cardiovascular Health

Maintaining a healthy cardiovascular system prevents heart disease, stroke, and other related health issues. While lifestyle factors such as diet, exercise, and stress management play a significant role, herbal remedies can also support heart health.

Some of the most common herbal remedies for cardiovascular health include:

Hawthorn

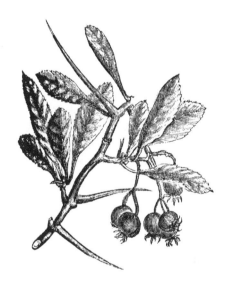

Hawthorn (Crataegus) is a small tree or shrub that belongs to the rose family. Known for strengthening and regulating the heart, this plant is an excellent choice for cardiovascular health. It contains flavonoids, which are potent antioxidants that help to protect the heart and blood vessels from damage caused by free radicals.Hawthorn is renowned for enhancing circulation and reducing blood pressure by dilating blood vessels, facilitating improved blood flow throughout the body. This makes it a valuable option for individuals dealing with poor circulation or high blood pressure.

If you decide to consume it as tea, Hawthorn tea is made by steeping the leaves and flowers of the hawthorn plant in hot water. Tinctures are concentrated extracts of the herb that are taken orally. Capsules are a convenient way to take hawthorn, allowing for precise dosing.

Arjuna

Arjuna (Terminalia arjuna) is an Ayurvedic herb that protects the heart and blood vessels from oxidative damage caused by free radicals. It also contains compounds that help dilate blood vessels, improving blood flow and reducing blood pressure. The herb has also demonstrated its ability to diminish plaque accumulation in the arteries, contributing to lower cholesterol levels and a reduced risk of cardiovascular discase.

Arjuna can be taken as a tea, tincture, or capsule form. It is important to note that Arjuna may interact with certain medications, such as blood thinners and beta-blockers. Therefore, speak with a healthcare provider before taking Arjuna to ensure its safety for your health needs.

Ginkgo Biloba

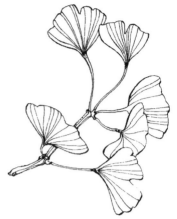

The benefits of Ginkgo Biloba stem from its rich content of flavonoids and terpenoids, which are potent antioxidants that protect cells from damage caused by free radicals. Ginkgo Biloba can help deliver essential nutrients and oxygen to the body's organs, including the brain and heart, by improving blood flow.

Moreover, the anti-inflammatory properties of Ginkgo Biloba help reduce the risk of cardiovascular diseases by minimizing the inflammation that contributes to plaque buildup in the arteries. This, in turn, can help prevent conditions such as atherosclerosis and reduce the risk of heart attacks and strokes.

Ginkgo Biloba is commonly taken as an extract or in capsule form to ensure a standardized dose of its active compounds. The extract is often derived from the dried leaves of the Ginkgo tree and is available in various concentrations.

Garlic

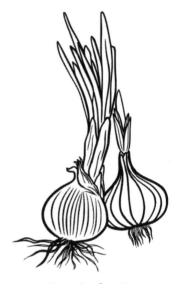

Garlic (Allium sativum), used for centuries in various cultures for its medicinal properties, is a potent natural remedy known for its numerous cardiovascular benefits. Why is it useful?

Lower Blood Pressure - Allicin in garlic helps to relax blood vessels, lowering blood pressure levels.

Reduce Cholesterol - Garlic has been shown to decrease cholesterol levels, further supporting heart health.

Decrease Heart Disease Risk - By reducing plaque buildup in the arteries, garlic helps to minimize the risk of heart disease.

You have several methods to incorporate garlic into your diet to experience its cardiovascular benefits:

Raw Garlic: You can add raw garlic to salads, sauces, and other dishes for added flavor and nutrition.

- Cooked Garlic: You may use cooked garlic in soups, stews, and other dishes to enjoy its health benefits.

- Supplements: You can consume garlic supplements or tablets to ensure consistent intake.

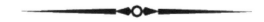

Recipes

Hawthorn Berry Tea

Ingredients:

- 2 tablespoons dried hawthorn berries

- 2 cups boiling water

- Honey or lemon to taste (optional)

Instructions:

1. Place dried hawthorn berries in a teapot or heat-proof pitcher.

2. Pour the boiling water over the berries.

3. Steep for 15 to 20 minutes.

4. Strain the tea into a cup.

5. Add honey or lemon to taste, if desired.

6. Drink 2-3 times daily.

Prep time: 25 minutes

Tips: Always use high-quality dried hawthorn berries for the best flavor and health benefits. Be patient and allow the tea to steep fully before drinking.

Garlic and Ginger Infused Honey

We have just explored the beneficial properties of garlic for cardiovascular health. Conversely, ginger is a powerful antioxidant and anti-inflammatory agent that can prevent heart and blood vessel damage.

Ingredients:

- 1 cup raw honey

- 4 cloves of garlic, peeled and crushed

- 2 inches of fresh ginger root, sliced

Instructions:

1. Place the crushed garlic and sliced ginger in a mason jar.

2. Pour raw honey over the garlic and ginger, making sure they are completely covered.

3. Seal the jar and allow the mixture to infuse for at least a week in a cool, dark place.

4. Take a teaspoon of this infused honey daily.

Prep time: 7 days

Tips: It is better to use raw, unprocessed honey for this recipe to maximize health benefits. If the flavor of garlic is too strong for you, you can increase the amount of honey.

Heart-Healthy Turmeric Latte

Cinnamon is known for reducing high blood cholesterol and triglyceride levels. Turmeric contains a compound called curcumin, which has anti-inflammatory and antioxidant effects. These properties may protect against heart disease by reducing inflammation and oxidative stress.

Ingredients:

- 2 cups of almond milk

- 1 teaspoon turmeric powder

- 1/2 teaspoon cinnamon powder

- A pinch of black pepper

- Honey to taste

Instructions:

1. Warm the almond milk in a saucepan.

2. Stir in the turmeric, cinnamon, and black pepper.

3. Heat the mixture for 5 minutes on low heat.

4. Pour the latte into a cup, add honey to taste, and stir well.

5. Drink this latte once daily.

Prep time: 10 minutes

Tips: Adding black pepper increases the bioavailability of curcumin, the active ingredient in turmeric. Always add a pinch of it when consuming turmeric.

Flaxseed Oatmeal

Flaxseeds are a rich source of omega-3 fatty acids, specifically alpha-linolenic acid (ALA), which possess anti-inflammatory properties and help prevent the hardening of arteries. Furthermore, their high dietary fiber content aids in lowering levels of LDL (bad) cholesterol, thereby reducing the risk of heart disease. LDL stands for low-density lipoprotein, which is often referred to as "bad" cholesterol. Excess LDL cholesterol can contribute to plaque buildup in the arteries, increasing the risk of heart disease. Maintaining healthy levels of LDL cholesterol is essential for cardiovascular health.

Ingredients:

- 1 cup of oats

- 2 cups of water or almond milk

- 2 tablespoons ground flaxseeds

- Fresh berries and nuts for topping

Instructions:

1. In a saucepan, bring the water or almond milk to a boil.

2. Add the oats and simmer until they are cooked.

3. Stir in the ground flaxseeds.

4. Serve in a bowl and top with fresh berries and nuts.

Prep time: 15 minutes

Tips: Flaxseeds are best consumed ground as whole flaxseeds may pass undigested through your body. Also, you can simply add them to your dishes, such as salads, smoothies, or yogurts, for an extra nutritional punch. Don't heat flaxseeds, as it can destroy their beneficial compounds.

Diabetes Management

Diabetes management involves monitoring blood sugar levels, consuming a healthy diet, and staying physically active. When combined with conventional medications and lifestyle changes, herbal remedies can be a beneficial supplement to a comprehensive diabetes control plan.

Fenugreek

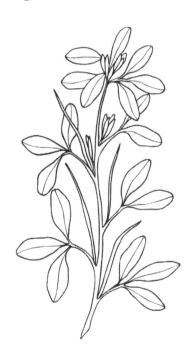

Fenugreek, scientifically known as Trigonella foenum-graecum, is an aromatic herb that has carved out a niche for itself both in culinary and medicinal traditions worldwide. Native to the Mediterranean region, Middle East, and Asia, it has been used for thousands of years to flavor food and remedy a variety of health conditions.

The golden seeds, with their nutty, slightly bitter flavor, are what we most often associate with fenugreek, but its leaves, too, are used both as a culinary ingredient and therapeutic agent.

Fenugreek has been used traditionally to enhance lactation in breastfeeding women and to alleviate digestive problems such as loss of appetite, upset stomach, and constipation.

However, fenugreek's potent antidiabetic properties are what set it apart in the realm of herbal medicine. The herb has shown promise in the management of both type 1 and type 2 diabetes. Fenugreek seeds are rich in dietary fiber, which can slow down the digestion of carbohydrates and hence, sugar absorption in the blood, leading to a gradual and controlled release of glucose.

Research also points towards the presence of an amino acid called 4-hydroxyisoleucine in fenugreek, which can stimulate the secretion of insulin, the hormone that regulates blood sugar levels. Studies have found that the consumption of fenugreek seeds, soaked in hot water, shows a significant effect in lowering blood glucose levels in people with diabetes.

In addition to its direct blood sugar-controlling effects, fenugreek may also assist with other conditions associated with diabetes, such as high cholesterol levels and heart disease, thanks to its antioxidant and lipid-lowering properties.

Despite the promising research, it's important to remember that while fenugreek may aid in diabetes management, it should not be used as a replacement for conventional treatment methods. It's crucial to consult a healthcare provider before incorporating fenugreek or any other herbal remedy into a treatment plan for diabetes or any other health condition.

Bitter Melon

Bitter melon, also known as bitter gourd or Momordica charantia, can potentially lower blood sugar levels by increasing insulin sensitivity and promoting glucose metabolism. According to a study from 2018, bitter melon compounds may help reduce blood glucose levels.

The researchers found changes in receptors that may be involved in the body's uptake and use of glucose when rats were fed a diet that included bitter melon leaf. Bitter melon can be consumed in various forms, such as juice, extract, or capsules.

Gymnema

Gymnema (Gymnema sylvestre), also known as Gurmar, is an Ayurvedic herb used in Indian traditional medicine for centuries to help regulate blood sugar levels and reduce sugar cravings.

This herb is believed to work by blocking the absorption of sugar in the intestines and supporting insulin production, helping to maintain healthy blood sugar levels.

Cinnamon

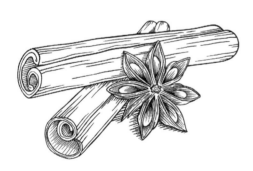

Cinnamon, derived from the bark of trees in the Cinnamomum family, is a spice renowned worldwide for its distinctive aroma and flavor. Used in both sweet and savory dishes, it's a staple in many global cuisines. However, cinnamon's potential extends beyond the kitchen. For centuries, it has held a significant place in traditional medicine, recognized for its array of potential health benefits. Among these, its role in diabetes management is particularly noteworthy.

Diabetes, specifically type 2, is a widespread health condition characterized by high blood sugar levels due to insulin resistance or the inability of the pancreas to produce enough insulin. Modern research has found that cinnamon may aid in managing this condition.

Cinnamon contains a compound called cinnamaldehyde, which gives the spice its flavor and aroma. More importantly, cinnamaldehyde and other compounds present in cinnamon are thought to have insulin-mimicking properties. This means they can potentially help regulate blood sugar levels, a critical factor in diabetes management.

Several studies suggest that consuming cinnamon may help lower blood sugar levels and improve insulin sensitivity in individuals with type 2 diabetes or prediabetes. The spice seems to reduce the speed at which the stomach empties after meals, reducing the rise in blood sugar after eating.

Cinnamon's potential effect on lipid profiles is also noteworthy. Some research indicates that it may help decrease total cholesterol, LDL cholesterol, and triglycerides, all of which, when elevated, are risk factors for diabetes complications.

To incorporate cinnamon into a diabetes management plan, it can be sprinkled on whole grain toast, mixed into oatmeal, or added to herbal teas for a flavorful twist. Cinnamon supplements are also available, but it's crucial to consult a healthcare professional before starting any supplement regimen.

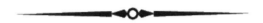

Recipes

Fenugreek Seed Infusion

Ingredients:

- 1 tablespoon fenugreek seeds
- 2 cups of water

Instructions:

1. Soak the fenugreek seeds overnight in the water.

2. In the morning, strain the water into a glass.

3. Drink this water on an empty stomach.

Prep time: Overnight + 5 minutes

Tips: Fenugreek seeds can be found at health food stores or online. It's always best to consult with a healthcare provider before starting any new regimen, especially for those on medications, as fenugreek can interact with certain drugs.

Cinnamon and Ginger Tea

Ingredients:

- 1 inch of fresh ginger root, peeled and sliced
- 1 cinnamon stick
- 2 cups of water

Instructions:

1. Place the cinnamon stick and sliced ginger in a pot with the water.

2. Bring the mixture to a boil, then reduce to a simmer for 15-20 minutes.

3. Strain the tea into a mug, discarding the solids.

Prep time: 30 minutes

Tips: If you prefer a sweeter taste, you can add a small amount of stevia or monk fruit sweetener to the mixture. It's important to avoid using sugar or honey, as they can cause a spike in blood glucose levels.

Aloe Vera Smoothie

Aloe Vera contains phytosterols which have anti-hyperglycemic effects. It's also known for its anti-inflammatory benefits.

Ingredients:

- 2 tablespoons of fresh aloe vera gel

- 1 cup of unsweetened almond milk

- A handful of blueberries

- 1 tablespoon of chia seeds

Instructions:

1. Scoop out fresh aloe vera gel from the leaf.

2. Put the aloe vera gel, almond milk, blueberries, and chia seeds into a blender.

3. Blend until smooth.

Prep time: 15 minutes

Tips: Always use fresh aloe vera gel from the plant. It's also recommended to check if you're allergic to aloe vera before ingesting it.

Bitter Gourd Juice

Ingredients:

- 1 medium-sized bitter gourd

- 1/2 a lemon

- A pinch of pink Himalayan salt

Instructions:

1. Wash and chop the bitter gourd, removing the seeds.

2. Extract the juice with a juicer.

3. Squeeze the lemon into the juice and add a pinch of salt.

4. Mix well and drink.

Prep time: 15 minutes

Tips: Bitter gourd juice can be strong and bitter. It's best to start with a small quantity and gradually increase. Add more lemon juice or a little water to dilute if the bitterness is too much.

Chapter Two

Specialized Chronic Conditions

Immune Support

A robust immune system is essential for maintaining good health and preventing infections, illnesses, and diseases. Factors like stress, lack of sleep, poor diet, and insufficient exercise can all weaken the immune system, making it more susceptible to health issues. Some herbs help keep our immune system in good shape; let's see which ones.

Oregano

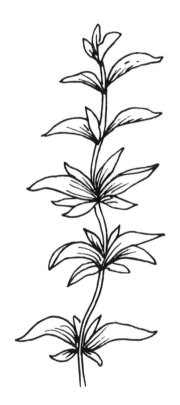

Oregano, known scientifically as Origanum vulgare, is a perennial herb native to the Mediterranean region and a staple in Italian and Greek cuisine. Its name comes from the Greek words "oros," meaning mountain, and "ganos," meaning joy. Beyond its gastronomic delights, oregano has been lauded for its healing properties since ancient times.

Let's explore some of the most prevalent uses of oregano as a herbal remedy, particularly its potent role in immune system support.

Digestive Disorders – As a rich source of dietary fiber, oregano can help improve digestive health by facilitating healthy bowel movements and preventing constipation. Traditional medicine also uses oregano to alleviate symptoms of indigestion, bloating, and heartburn.

Respiratory Conditions – Oregano has been used in traditional medicine to relieve symptoms associated with respiratory ailments, such as cough, cold, and bronchitis, due to its expectorant properties which help clear mucus from the lungs.

Pain Relief – With its anti-inflammatory and analgesic properties, oregano can offer relief from muscle aches and pains. It is also used topically to alleviate the discomfort of conditions such as arthritis and joint pain.

Now, let's focus on the star feature of this herb – its ability to enhance the immune system. Oregano is packed with antioxidants, substances that can neutralize harmful free radicals in the body. This is mainly due to two powerful compounds it contains: carvacrol and thymol.

Carvacrol has been studied for its antimicrobial properties that can help the body fend off infection. Meanwhile, thymol, a natural fungicide with antiseptic properties, can support the immune system by protecting against toxins.

Many people use oregano oil, a concentrated form of the herb, as a natural remedy during cold and flu season. It's thought to help prevent infections, thanks to its antiviral and antibacterial qualities, while also promoting a healthy inflammatory response.

In addition, preliminary research suggests that oregano may stimulate the production of white blood cells, the body's primary defense mechanism against pathogens.

Overall, whether sprinkled on your favorite dishes or used in its concentrated oil form, oregano offers substantial potential in boosting immunity and maintaining overall health. Nevertheless, as with all herbal remedies, it's crucial to consult with a healthcare provider before starting any new treatment regimen.

Elderberry

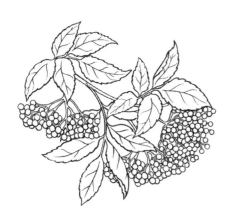

Elderberry (Sambucus nigra) is a powerful antioxidant with antiviral properties. Rich in vitamins A, B, and C, as well as flavonoids and anthocyanins, elderberry provides essential nutrients that support the body's natural defense mechanisms. The high antioxidant content of elderberry also helps to neutralize harmful free radicals that can damage cells and contribute to chronic diseases.

There are several ways to incorporate elderberry into your daily routine for immune support. Elderberry syrup is a popular option, often mixed with honey to create a pleasant-tasting remedy that can be taken on its own or added to tea or yogurt.

Elderberry gummies and lozenges offer a convenient and portable way to enjoy the benefits of elderberry, especially for those who prefer not to take liquid supplements. Additionally, elderberry teas and extracts can be found in health food stores or prepared at home using dried elderberries.

Andrographis

If you're looking for an effective way to boost your immunity functions, look no further than Andrographis (Andrographis paniculata). Dubbed the "King of Bitters" due to its flavor profile, Ayurvedic and traditional Chinese medicine have utilized this herb's immune-boosting and anti-inflammatory capabilities since ancient times.

Incorporating Andorgraphis into your wellness regime has never been easier, with many options available with varying taste preferences. Capsules and tinctures offer convenience and potent delivery methods, while teas provide a more relaxing experience.

Reishi Mushroom

Often called the "mushroom of immortality," reishi mushroom (Ganoderma lucidum) has been a staple in Traditional Chinese Medicine for centuries due to its powerful immune-boosting properties. As a renowned adaptogen, reishi helps the body adapt to stress and supports a healthy immune response.

Reishi is a powerful immune booster! It's rich in antioxidants and beta-glucans that strengthen your immune system. It increases the activity of white blood cells and promotes the production of cytokines, which are essential for a strong immune response. Reishi also improves energy levels, reduces inflammation, and supports overall well-being. You can add reishi to your routine in powder, capsule, or tincture form to give your immune system a superhero boost!

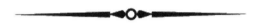

Recipes

Immune-Boosting Herbal Tea

Ingredients:

- 1 teaspoon dried Echinacea

- 1/2 teaspoon grated ginger

- 1/2 teaspoon turmeric powder

- 1 slice of lemon

- Honey (optional, for taste)

- 1 cup of water

Instructions:

1. Bring the water to a boil in a pot.

2. Add Echinacea, ginger, and turmeric.

3. Reduce heat and let simmer for 10-15 minutes.

4. Strain the tea into a cup, add the lemon slice, and sweeten with honey if desired.

Prep Time: 20 minutes.

Tips: Consume this tea 2-3 times a week for maximum benefits.

Elderberry Syrup

Ingredients:

- 1 cup dried elderberries

- 4 cups of water

- 1 cup of raw honey

Instructions:

1. Bring the water to a boil, and add elderberries.

2. Reduce heat and let simmer for about 45 minutes or until the liquid has reduced by half.

3. Mash the elderberries to release the remaining juice and strain the mixture into a glass jar.

4. Let the liquid cool and then add honey and stir until well combined.

5. Store in the refrigerator.

Prep Time: 1 hour 10 minutes.

Tips: Take 1-2 tablespoons daily for immune support.

Herbal Immune Support Gummies

Ingredients:

- 1/2 cup Echinacea herbal tea

- 1/2 cup rosehip syrup

- 1/4 cup honey

- 1/4 cup unflavored gelatin

Instructions:

1. Brew the Echinacea tea and let it cool.

2. Combine the tea, rosehip syrup, and honey in a saucepan and warm over low heat.

3. Sprinkle the gelatin over the liquid and stir until the gelatin completely dissolves.

4. Pour the mixture into silicone molds and refrigerate until set (about 2-3 hours).

Prep Time: 3 hours 30 minutes.

Tips: These gummies can be stored in an airtight container in the refrigerator for up to two weeks.

Astragalus Garlic Soup

Ingredients:

- 2 Astragalus roots

- 6 cloves of garlic

- 1 onion

- 2 carrots

- 1 cup of chopped celery

- Salt and pepper to taste

- 6 cups of water

Instructions:

1. Saute onions, garlic, carrots, and celery in a large pot until onions are translucent.

2. Add water and astragalus roots.

3. Bring to a boil and then lower heat to simmer for about 1-2 hours.

4. Remove the astragalus roots.

5. Season the soup with salt and pepper to taste and serve warm.

Prep Time: 2 hours 30 minutes.

Tips: This soup is perfect for cold winter days and can be stored in the refrigerator for up to a week.

Lemon Balm and Ginger Infused Honey

Ingredients:

- 1 cup of raw honey

- 1/4 cup of fresh lemon balm leaves

- 2 tablespoons of freshly grated ginger

Instructions:

1. Place the lemon balm leaves and grated ginger in a jar.

2. Pour honey over the herbs and ensure they are completely covered.

3. Place the jar in a sunny window and let it infuse for at least two weeks, turning the jar over every couple of days.

4. After two weeks, strain the honey into a clean jar.

Prep Time: 2 weeks and 20 minutes.

Tips: This infused honey is excellent for tea, on toast, or by the spoonful for a quick immune boost.

Liver and Kidney Health

Our liver and kidneys play essential roles in maintaining our overall health, with the liver responsible for detoxification, metabolism, and digestion and the kidneys filtering waste and balancing electrolytes in our bodies. Maintaining their performance is vital for health. Here, we'll discuss common herbs for liver and kidney health and a simple home recipe.

Parsley

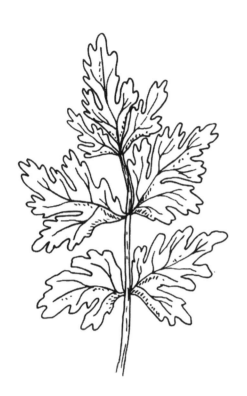

Parsley (Petroselinum crispum) is often relegated to the role of a simple garnish in many dishes. However, this vibrant, verdant herb, native to the Mediterranean, holds a significant position in the world of traditional medicine. Rich in vitamins and minerals, parsley offers more than just a visual appeal to your meals; it also presents a multitude of potential health benefits.

Commonly used applications of parsley include its use for digestive health, immune system support, and blood pressure management. The herb has long been reputed to improve digestion, bolster the immune system with its rich Vitamin C content, and help manage hypertension due to its diuretic properties.

However, one of the most notable uses of parsley in herbal medicine is its role in kidney health enhancement.

<u>Parsley for Kidney Health</u>

Parsley's natural diuretic properties have made it a favorite for kidney health. By promoting the production of urine, parsley can help the body eliminate excess fluid and flush out waste products from the kidneys. This action can contribute to maintaining kidney health by preventing the buildup of toxins in the body.

Traditional practices often recommend consuming parsley tea as a gentle yet effective diuretic. This is usually prepared by steeping fresh or dried parsley leaves in hot water. The result is a mildly flavored infusion believed to support the kidneys' function.

Moreover, the presence of certain compounds like flavonoids, terpenoids, and apigenin in parsley have been linked to kidney protective effects. Apigenin, in particular, is a natural antioxidant that has been studied for its potential role in protecting the kidneys from damage.

It's important to note that while parsley can offer support for kidney health, it shouldn't be considered a treatment for kidney diseases. If you are experiencing serious kidney problems, professional medical advice is imperative. Parsley should be used in moderation, as excessive consumption can have side effects. Always consult a healthcare provider before introducing any new herbal remedies into your regimen, particularly if you are pregnant, nursing, or on any medication.

Milk Thistle

Milk thistle (Silybum marianum) has garnered a reputation as a natural remedy due to its active compound, silymarin, which boasts antioxidant and anti-inflammatory properties. It is commonly used for the following purposes:

- Liver Support: Milk thistle is believed to support liver function and protect liver cells from damage caused by toxins, such as alcohol, pollutants, and certain medications.

- Liver Detoxification: It potentially enhances the liver's detoxification processes by promoting the production of enzymes involved in detoxification pathways.

- Liver Regeneration: Milk thistle supports the regeneration of liver tissue and encourages the growth of new liver cells.

- Liver Conditions: It is often used as a complementary approach for liver-related conditions such as cirrhosis, hepatitis (viral or alcoholic), fatty liver disease, and liver damage caused by certain medications.

- Gallbladder Health: Milk thistle may assist in improving gallbladder function and supporting bile production, which aids in the digestion and absorption of fats.

- Antioxidant Effects: Silymarin in milk thistle has antioxidant properties that can protect liver cells from oxidative stress and damage caused by free radicals.

Milk thistle come in various forms, including capsules, tablets, liquid extracts, and powders.

Dandelion

Dandelion (Taraxacum officinale) is a humble plant often dismissed as a mere weed. However, it is a potent natural remedy with numerous benefits for both liver and kidney health.

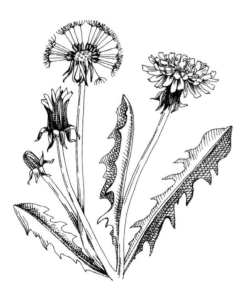

The root of the dandelion plant has been found to support liver function by promoting bile production, which aids the detoxification process. Bile is essential for breaking down fats and eliminating toxins from the liver, and dandelion root helps to stimulate its production. Additionally, dandelion root has potent anti-inflammatory properties, which can help alleviate liver inflammation and reduce the risk of liver damage.

On the other hand, dandelion leaves have natural diuretic properties, making them an excellent option for promoting kidney health. Diuretics help to increase urine output, which can assist in flushing out excess fluids, waste, and toxins from the body. This is particularly beneficial for individuals who suffer from kidney problems, as it helps reduce the kidneys' workload.

Drinking dandelion tea is a popular way to enjoy its health benefits, and it can be brewed using the dried leaves or roots of the plant. Dandelion tinctures and capsules are also commonly available at health food stores. If you want to try dandelion tea, here's a simple recipe:

Ingredients:

- 1 cup of fresh dandelion leaves (or 2 tablespoons of dried dandelion leaves)

- 2 cups of water

- Optional: sweetener of your choice (such as honey or stevia)

Instructions:

1. Rinse the dandelion leaves thoroughly to remove any dirt or debris.

2. Bring the water to a boil in a small pot.

3. Add the dandelion leaves to the boiling water and let it simmer for about 5 minutes.

4. Remove the pot from heat and let the tea steep for 5 minutes.

5. Strain the tea to remove the dandelion leaves.

6. If desired, add sweetener.

7. Serve the dandelion tea hot or chilled.

Note: Make sure that the dandelions you use for tea are from a safe and pesticide-free source. If you are not sure about foraging for dandelions, it's best to purchase dried leaves from a reputable source or use dandelion tea bags available in stores.aggiunto io

Turmeric

Turmeric (Curcuma longa), known for its vibrant yellow color and unique flavor, is also a potent liver and kidney supporter. Its active compound, curcumin, boasts antioxidant and anti-inflammatory properties that help protect liver cells and support detoxification. Also, turmeric may help prevent kidney damage caused by oxidative stress.

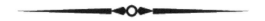

Recipes

Dandelion Root Tea

Ingredients:

- 1 tablespoon dried dandelion root

- 2 cups of water

- Honey or lemon to taste (optional)

Instructions:

1. Place the dandelion root in a saucepan and add the water.

2. Bring to a boil, then lower the heat and let it simmer for about 15 minutes.

3. Strain the tea into a cup, add honey or lemon if desired, and serve.

Prep Time: 20 minutes

Tips: Dandelion root can be bitter, so feel free to adjust the amount according to your taste preference.

Milk Thistle Seed Tincture

Ingredients:

- 1 cup of milk thistle seeds

- 2 cups of high-proof alcohol (like vodka)

Instructions:

1. Crush the milk thistle seeds lightly to release their oils.

2. Place the crushed seeds in a glass jar, and cover them with the alcohol.

3. Seal the jar tightly and leave it in a cool, dark place for about 4 weeks, shaking it every few days.

4. After 4 weeks, strain the tincture into another jar, and it's ready to use.

Prep Time: 4 weeks

Tips: The standard dosage for a tincture like this is generally 1-2 ml, taken 3 times per day. Please consult with a healthcare provider for accurate dosage recommendations.

Nettle and Parsley Infused Water

Nettle and parsley are two herbs traditionally used for kidney health. Nettle has diuretic properties, which can help flush out toxins from the kidneys. Parsley is also believed to have similar properties and is often used to help control kidney stones.

Ingredients:

- 1 tablespoon dried nettle leaves

- 1 tablespoon dried parsley

- 1 liter of water

Instructions:

1. Boil the water in a pot.

2. Add the dried nettle leaves and dried parsley.

3. Lower the heat and let it simmer for about 15 minutes.

4. Strain the water and let it cool.

Prep Time: 25 minutes

Tips: You can drink this infused water throughout the day to help support your kidney health.

Cranberry Juice

Cranberries have long been associated with kidney and urinary tract health. They contain compounds called proanthocyanidins, which can help prevent bacteria from sticking to the walls of the urinary tract.

Ingredients:

- 2 cups of fresh cranberries

- 4 cups of water

- Honey to taste (optional)

Instructions:

1. Rinse the cranberries and place them in a pot with the water.

2. Bring to a boil, then reduce the heat and let it simmer for about 20 minutes until the cranberries have burst.

3. Let the mixture cool a bit, then puree it in a blender until smooth.

4. Strain the juice into a pitcher, pressing on the solids to extract as much juice as possible.

5. If desired, add honey to taste. Serve chilled or over ice.

Prep Time: 35 minutes

Tips: This cranberry juice can be stored in the fridge and consumed daily. Store-bought cranberry juice often contains added sugars, so making your own is a healthier alternative.

Memory and Cognitive Function

Cognitive function includes a range of mental abilities such as memory, attention, problem-solving, and language skills. Various factors, including age, stress, lack of sleep, and certain health conditions, can negatively impact these abilities, leading to forgetfulness, difficulty concentrating, and slowed thinking.

On the other hand, memory issues are related explicitly to storing, retaining, and recalling information. While it's normal to experience occasional forgetfulness, significant memory problems can interfere with daily life and may be a sign of more severe conditions, like dementia or Alzheimer's disease.

When it comes to cognitive health and memory enhancement, many individuals turn to nature for natural solutions. By exploring the realm of herbal remedies, you can discover a natural and holistic path to nurture your cognitive health and elevate your memory capabilities.

Rosemary

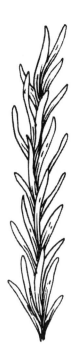

But the benefits of rosemary don't stop there; even this herb's aroma can positively affect our cognitive function. Studies have shown that simply inhaling the scent of rosemary can enhance concentration, speed up cognitive processing, and improve memory retention.

There are various methods for enjoying the benefits of rosemary. A straightforward approach is to incorporate fresh or dried rosemary into your cooking. The herb pairs well with many foods, including roasted vegetables, soups, and meats.

For a more concentrated dose, consider using rosemary essential oil. A few drops can be added to a diffuser to fill your living or workspace with its refreshing scent, providing cognitive benefits as you go about your day. Alternatively, add a few drops to a warm bath or massage oil for a relaxing and rejuvenating treatment. As always, it's essential to use essential oils safely – they should typically be diluted before use, and always do a patch test on your skin to check for any adverse reactions.

Rosemary supplements are also available, offering a convenient way to enjoy the herb's benefits. However, as with any supplement, consult a healthcare provider before starting a new regimen, especially if you have any underlying health conditions.

Bacopa monnieri

Bacopa monnieri, often known as Brahmi in traditional Ayurvedic medicine, is a potent plant with a long history of use as a brain enhancer. In modern science, the anecdotal claims about Bacopa monnieri are gaining validation.

This perennial herb contains bacosides, active chemical compounds that are thought to work by healing damaged neurons in the brain, which can become weakened due to factors like stress, aging, and environmental toxins. Bacopa monnieri may help enhance neural communication, improving cognitive functions such as memory, attention, and reasoning.

Bacopa monnieri may also have neuroprotective qualities, according to research. This means it may help protect the brain from damage and degeneration, potentially improving long-term brain health.

Ashwagandha

Ashwagandha, an essential herb in Ayurvedic medicine, is steeped in centuries of use and respect for its incredible health benefits, notably its potential to bolster brain function, including memory. This herb, whose botanical name is Withania somnifera, is also known as "Indian ginseng" due to its rejuvenating properties.

One of the compelling aspects of Ashwagandha's action on the brain is its power to mitigate memory and cognitive dysfunction associated with neurodegenerative diseases such as Alzheimer's and Parkinson's. This potential stems from its antioxidant activity, which combats oxidative stress, a significant contributor to neuronal damage in these diseases.

Ashwagandha is thought to improve brain plasticity, namely its ability to change and adapt. This is critical for memory and learning processes. It may also increase nerve cell proliferation, improving brain communication and cognitive function.

Regarding practical application, Ashwagandha is versatile and may be integrated into your daily routine in various ways. Ashwagandha powder can be mixed into your morning smoothie, breakfast bowl, or warm milk before bed. It is also available in capsule and tincture form if you wish to try a more convenient approach.

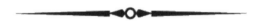

Recipes

Ginkgo Biloba and Green Tea

Ingredients:

- 1 tsp of dried Ginkgo Biloba leaves
- 1 tsp of organic green tea
- 1 tsp of honey
- 1 cup of boiling water

Instructions:

1. Combine the Ginkgo Biloba leaves and green tea in a teapot or mug.

2. Pour boiling water over the leaves and steep for 3-5 minutes.

3. Strain the mixture and add honey for taste. Enjoy warm.

Preparation Time: 10 minutes

Tips: Choose high-quality, organic tea leaves for a healthier and more beneficial brew. Drink this tea in the morning as Ginkgo Biloba can stimulate and might interfere with sleep if consumed in the evening.

Rosemary Infused Olive Oil

Ingredients:

- 2 cups of extra virgin olive oil
- 3-4 sprigs of fresh rosemary

Instructions:

1. Wash the rosemary sprigs and let them dry completely.

2. Place the dried rosemary sprigs into a clean glass jar.

3. Pour the olive oil into the jar, fully submerging the rosemary.

4. Seal the jar and store it in a cool, dark place for two weeks, shaking it once every few days.

5. After two weeks, strain out the rosemary and use your infused oil as you please.

Preparation Time: 2 weeks steeping time

Tips: You can use this oil for cooking or as a salad dressing.

Bacopa Monnieri Tincture

Ingredients:

- 1 cup of Bacopa Monnieri (fresh or dried)
- 2 cups of high-proof alcohol (like vodka)

Instructions:

1. Place Bacopa Monnieri in a clean mason jar.

2. Pour alcohol over the herb until it's completely covered.

3. Seal the jar tightly and store it in a cool, dark place.

4. Shake the jar daily for the first few days, then at least once a week for the remaining weeks.

5. Strain the mixture using cheesecloth after 4-6 weeks and store the liquid in a clean, glass container.

Preparation Time: 4-6 weeks

Tips: You can take a dropper full of this tincture daily. Remember that Bacopa Monnieri acts gradually, so you may see benefits in memory and cognitive performance after a few weeks.

Sage Herbal Honey

Ingredients:

- 1 cup of fresh sage leaves
- 1 cup of raw honey

Instructions:

1. Place the fresh sage leaves in a glass jar.

2. Pour honey over the sage leaves until they are fully covered.

3. Stir the mixture to remove air bubbles and ensure the leaves are fully coated.

4. Cover the jar and let it sit in a cool, dark place for two weeks. 5. Stir or turn the jar upside down every few days to keep the leaves coated in honey.

5. After two weeks, strain the mixture to remove the leaves and store your sage-infused honey in a clean jar.

Preparation Time: 14 days

Tips: You can consume this herbal honey directly or add it to tea or warm water. This is a sweet and easy way to incorporate sage into your diet and support your cognitive function. Remember, herbal remedies take time to show their effects, so patience is key to experiencing the full benefits.

Respiratory Health

Respiratory health is a vital aspect of our overall well-being that can often be undermined by common conditions such as bronchitis, asthma, allergies, and even the common cold or flu. These conditions can lead to symptoms like coughing, wheezing, shortness of breath, and general discomfort. Fortunately, nature has provided us with many herbs to support our respiratory health, relieving these symptoms and enhancing our lung function.

Eucalyptus

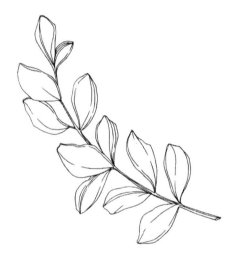

The secret of Eucalyprus lies in its leaves, which are rich in a compound known as eucalyptol. This constituent has the unique ability to thin out mucus and phlegm that often congest our respiratory tracts, making it easier for us to breathe. It's like nature's own decongestant. Eucalyptus is also a fierce defender against respiratory infections, for it has antimicrobial properties that can help eliminate pathogens, reducing the risk of further aggravating the respiratory system.

Boil a handful of eucalyptus leaves in water, remove from heat, and then cover your head with a towel, leaning over the pot to trap the steam. Breathe in the eucalyptus-infused steam to help clear your nasal passages and lungs. Eucalyptus essential oil can be added to a diffuser or warm bath. Another effective way to use eucalyptus is to make a homemade chest rub. See the recipe in the following section.

Licorice Root

With a sweet and slightly bitter flavor, licorice root (Glycyrrhiza glabra) is more than just the primary ingredient in a well-loved candy. It has a long-standing history in various traditional medicine systems worldwide, from Ayurveda to Traditional Chinese Medicine.

Licorice root is known for its anti-inflammatory property, making it particularly beneficial for reducing inflammation in the respiratory tract, which can be a common symptom in conditions such as bronchitis, asthma, or even the common cold.

Licorice root is well-regarded for its demulcent qualities, providing soothing relief for irritated mucous membranes. This property makes it an excellent remedy for sore throats, as it can provide a protective coating that helps to relieve pain and irritation. Moreover, licorice root acts as an expectorant. It helps to loosen and clear mucus from the lungs and airways, further aiding in alleviating respiratory issues. This clearing effect can help to relieve congestion and make coughs more productive.

Thyme

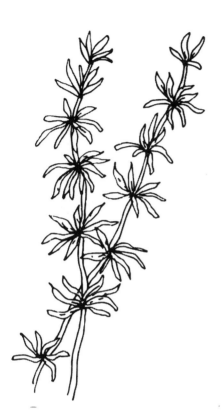

Thyme, scientifically known as Thymus vulgaris, is a remarkable herb that often goes unnoticed despite its potent benefits for lung health. Packed with essential vitamins C and A, along with minerals like copper, iron, and manganese, thyme offers a wealth of nutritional value. Its exceptional antiseptic and antibiotic properties set thyme apart, making it a valuable ally in addressing respiratory problems.

These properties stem from its rich content of antiseptic compounds, enabling thyme to combat respiratory infections effectively. By inhibiting the growth of bacteria, fungi, and viruses that contribute to respiratory issues, thyme proves itself as a reliable companion during the cold and flu season.

Thyme is also helpful as an expectorant. That's significant because thinning mucus in the lungs is crucial to alleviating congestion and restoring easy breathing. In addition, the calming effects of thyme on a cough might make it less bothersome and easier on the throat.

Recipes

Eucalyptus Chest Rub

Ingredients:

- 15 drops of eucalyptus essential oil

- 1/4 cup of coconut oil

- 1/4 cup of beeswax pellets

Instructions:

1. Melt the beeswax and coconut oil in a double boiler.

2. Remove from heat and let it cool slightly.

3. Stir in the eucalyptus essential oil.

4. Pour the mixture into a small jar and allow it to cool completely.

5. Rub on the chest and upper back to help clear the respiratory tract.

Preparation Time: 25 minutes

Tips: Always perform a patch test before using the chest rub, as some people may be sensitive to eucalyptus oil.

Thyme Tea

Ingredients:

- 2 teaspoons of dried thyme

- 2 cups of boiling water

- Honey or lemon juice to taste

Instructions:

1. Place dried thyme in a teapot or cup.

2. Pour boiling water over the thyme.

3. Allow it to steep for 10-15 minutes.

4. Strain, add honey or lemon juice if desired, and drink warm.

Preparation Time: 20 minutes

Tips: You can also use fresh thyme. Just double the amount to get the same potency as the dried version.

Mullein Leaf Steam Inhalation

Mullein is a go-to herb for tackling respiratory issues. It's thought to have anti-inflammatory, expectorant, and antibacterial properties that can help soothe the lungs and airways and loosen up phlegm.

Ingredients:

- A handful of dried mullein leaves

- A large bowl of boiling water

Instructions:

1. Place the mullein leaves in a large bowl.

2. Pour boiling water over the leaves.

3. Lean over the bowl and cover your head with a towel, creating a steam tent.

4. Breathe deeply for 5-10 minutes.

Preparation Time: 15 minutes

Tips: Be sure to keep your face at a safe distance from the steam to avoid burns.

Ginger-Turmeric Honey Bomb

Ginger and turmeric are both widely known for their anti-inflammatory properties, and they also work as natural decongestants and antihistamines. They're packed with antioxidants that can help improve immune function and combat respiratory infections.

Ingredients:

- 3 tablespoons of freshly grated ginger
- 3 tablespoons of turmeric powder
- 1 cup of raw honey

Instructions:

1. Combine the grated ginger, turmeric powder, and honey in a small bowl.

2. Stir until all the ingredients are thoroughly mixed.

3. Store this honey bomb in a glass jar.

4. Take one tablespoon daily, or add it to your tea, toast, or smoothie.

Preparation Time: 10 minutes

Tips: Keep the mixture in a cool, dry place. It should last for several weeks.

Elderberry Syrup

Elderberries are high in vitamins A, B, and C and stimulate the immune system. They are often used to treat cold and flu symptoms, including coughs and congestion.

Ingredients:

- 1 cup of dried elderberries
- 4 cups of water
- 1 cup of raw honey

Instructions:

1. Put elderberries and water into a pot and bring to a boil.

2. Reduce heat and let it simmer for about 45 minutes to an hour until the liquid reduces by half.

3. Remove from heat and let it cool.

4. Mash the berries and strain the liquid.

5. Stir in honey and store the syrup in a glass bottle in the refrigerator.

6. Take 1-2 tablespoons daily.

Preparation Time: 1 hour 15

BOOK IV

HERBAL
FIRST AID

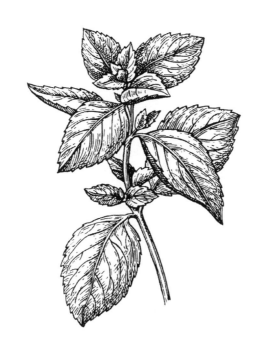

AMBER WHITMORE

Introduction

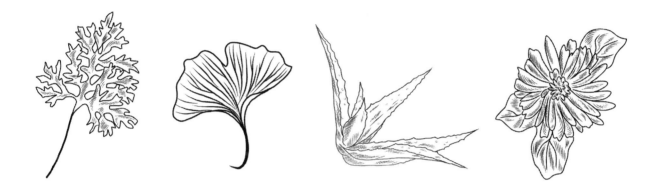

I always say there's a plant for every pinch and a flower for every folly. This book is all about first aid, the herbal way. You'd be surprised how many common ailments can be soothed with herbs.

All of us will encounter minor injuries and irritations throughout our lives, such as burns from accidentally touching a hot pan or bruises from bumping into furniture. Insect bites and stings can put a damper on an otherwise enjoyable day outdoors, and who can forget the discomfort of poison ivy or other skin irritants? Also, toothaches and gum issues can strike at the most inconvenient times, leaving us needing relief.

We will cover the basics of dealing with everyday injuries and irritations using herbal remedies. Each section will focus on a specific ailment type, providing a brief overview, recommended herbal treatments, and helpful application tips. By the end of this book, you'll have a solid foundation in herbal first aid, equipped with the knowledge to confidently address these common issues using nature's medicine cabinet.

Chapter One

Herbal First Aid - Part I

Burns and Sunburns

Burns and sunburns are common injuries that can occur due to various factors, such as exposure to heat, chemicals, electricity, or radiation. Sunburns, in particular, are caused by overexposure to the sun's ultraviolet (UV) rays. Immediate care is crucial in treating these injuries to alleviate pain, prevent infection, and promote healing.

Calendula

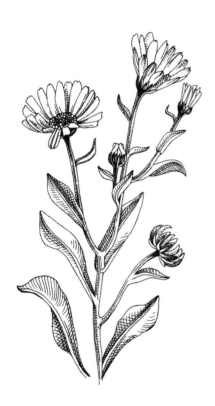

Calendula, also known as pot marigold, is a highly regarded plant in herbal medicine. This annual or biennial plant features bright orange or yellow flowers used in medicinal, culinary, and cosmetic applications for centuries.

Calendula offers substantial benefits for burns and sunburns. Its flowers are rich in flavonoids and carotenoids, both potent antioxidants that help speed up the healing process of burns. Additionally, Calendula has anti-inflammatory properties, which can help reduce swelling and pain associated with these types of skin injuries.

The preparation and application of Calendula for burns and sunburns involve using the plant's flowers. A simple remedy is a Calendula poultice. To make a soothing poultice for a burn, start by soaking fresh or dried flowers of the herb in hot water. Allow them to steep until a thick paste forms. Once ready, gently apply the paste directly onto the burn and cover it with a clean bandage.

This poultice can provide natural relief and support the healing process of the burn. Remember to change the poultice regularly and seek medical attention for severe burns.

For a more versatile remedy, Calendula-infused oil can be prepared. This involves steeping dried Calendula flowers in a carrier oil, such as olive or sweet almond oil, for several weeks. After straining the flowers, the resulting oil can be used directly on the skin or as a base for salves or creams.

Aloe Vera

Aloe Vera, a hero in the world of herbal remedies! A member of the succulent family, Aloe Vera is characterized by its thick, fleshy leaves that contain a clear, gel-like substance. This gel is the main component used in burn and sunburn treatment.

The efficacy of Aloe Vera in treating burns and sunburns is attributed to its anti-inflammatory and healing properties. It contains active components such as aloin and aloesin, which have been shown to reduce inflammation and alleviate pain. Aloe Vera is truly remarkable for its ability to support skin healing, especially when it comes to treating burns. It contains a special carbohydrate called acemannan, which works wonders in promoting the growth and repair of skin cells. So if you're dealing with a burn, Aloe Vera can be your go-to natural remedy for soothing and speeding up the healing process.

The preparation and application of Aloe Vera for burns and sunburns is easy. The most direct method involves cutting a leaf from the Aloe Vera plant, slicing it open to reveal the gel, and applying this directly to the affected area. Doing so provides a cooling effect and immediate relief from pain and inflammation.

An Aloe Vera salve can be prepared for a more refined and longer-lasting remedy. This involves extracting the gel from approximately two Aloe Vera leaves and mixing it with a quarter cup of melted coconut oil. Once cooled, this salve can be stored and applied to burns as needed. It combines Aloe Vera's healing properties and coconut oil's moisturizing effects, promoting swift and effective recovery.

Lavender

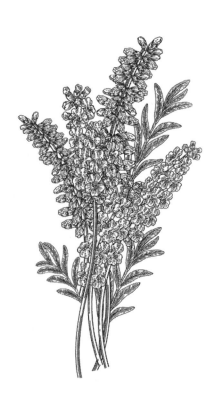

Lavender holds a prominent position in professional herbal medicine due to its wide-ranging therapeutic properties and ease of cultivation. This perennial plant, characterized by its purple flowers and silvery-green foliage, has been utilized in traditional medicine and aromatherapy for centuries.

Lavender is a highly effective remedy in the context of burns and sunburns. Its healing properties are mainly due to the essential oil extracted from its flowers, which contains compounds like linalool and linalyl acetate. These compounds have been studied for their antimicrobial, anti-inflammatory, and analgesic properties. This makes Lavender a potent herb for reducing inflammation, alleviating pain, and preventing infection in burns.

The preparation and application of Lavender for treating burns and sunburns involve using Lavender essential oil. It's crucial to remember that essential oils should never be applied undiluted directly to the skin. You can dilute a few drops of Lavender essential oil in a carrier oil, like coconut or jojoba oil, and apply it to the affected area for a simple, immediate burn remedy.

For a more complex and multi-purpose remedy, a Lavender-infused salve can be prepared. This involves blending Lavender essential oil with beeswax and carrier oil, heating until combined, then allowing the mixture to cool and solidify. This salve can be applied to burns, providing relief and promoting healing.

Recipes

<u>Aloe Vera Gel</u>

Ingredients:

- Fresh Aloe Vera leaf

Instructions:

1. Wash the Aloe Vera leaf thoroughly.

2. Cut off the spiky edges and peel off the skin on one side.

3. Scoop out the gel using a spoon and collect it in a clean container.

Prep Time: 10 minutes

Tips: You can store the remaining gel in a refrigerator for later use. Apply the gel gently onto the burn area several times a day.

<u>Lavender Oil Burn Spray</u>

Ingredients:

- 1 cup distilled water

- 10 drops Lavender Essential Oil

- Spray bottle

Instructions:

1. Fill the spray bottle with distilled water.

2. Add the lavender essential oil.

3. Shake well before each use.

Prep Time: 5 minutes

Tips: Spritz the mixture onto the affected area for pain relief and healing. Always do a patch test before applying essential oils to ensure you're not allergic.

<u>Plantain Poultice</u>

Plantain leaves (the common weed, not the banana-like fruit) are known for their natural anti-inflammatory and wound-healing properties. A poultice made from these leaves can soothe the pain of burns and promote skin recovery.

Ingredients:

- A handful of fresh Plantain leaves

- Water

Instructions:

1. Rinse the plantain leaves to remove any dirt or debris.

2. Crush the leaves with a little bit of water to create a paste. You can do this using a pestle and mortar.

3. Once you have a paste-like consistency, apply it directly to the burn.

Prep Time: 10 minutes

Tips: Replace the poultice when it gets warm. Use fresh plantain leaves for each application.

Cuts, Scrapes, and Bruises

These minor injuries are common, from scraped knees from childhood adventures to kitchen knife nicks while prepping dinner. But that doesn't mean they can't cause discomfort or take time to heal. And that's where the power of herbal remedies comes into play.

Yarrow

With its feathery leaves and clusters of white to pink flowers, Yarrow might seem unassuming at first glance, but it is an incredibly potent medicinal plant. Achillea millefolium, its scientific name, even alludes to the legendary Greek hero Achilles, who supposedly used it to treat wounds on the battlefield—so we're talking serious historical credibility here.

One of the most striking abilities of yarrow is its effectiveness in stopping bleeding. Applying crushed yarrow leaves can significantly slow down and stop bleeding, thanks to compounds like achilletin and achilleine, whether it's a fresh scrape or a nosebleed. This property, known as being hemostatic, has been noted and utilized by herbalists and healers for centuries.

But yarrow doesn't just stop there. It's also a natural anti-inflammatory, which means it can help reduce swelling in and around the wound. So whether you're dealing with insect bites, sprains, or recovering from surgery, yarrow has got your back.

Yarrow also has analgesic—or pain-relieving—properties. It helps numb the area and relieve discomfort, making it a triple threat in wound care. It's like nature's little first-aid kit wrapped in one charming, humble plant.

Hyssop

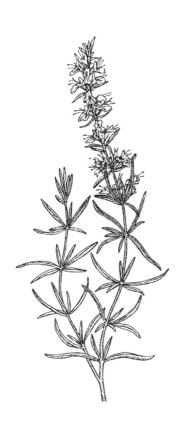

Hyssop, scientifically known as Hyssopus officinalis, is a flowering plant in the mint family, native to parts of Europe and the Middle East. Known for its vibrant, fragrant blossoms and bitter, aromatic leaves, hyssop has a storied history dating back to ancient times. It's been mentioned in biblical texts and used by traditional healers throughout the centuries.

Hyssop's utility in herbal medicine is diverse, with common uses including respiratory health support, as a digestive aid, and a calming agent for anxiety and stress. However, hyssop's potential as a skin care remedy, particularly for minor skin injuries such as cuts, bruises, and scrapes, deserves special attention.

Hyssop's antiseptic properties make it an excellent natural option for treating minor skin injuries. The herb's essential oil, when diluted properly, can be applied to cuts, scrapes, and bruises to clean the wound and potentially accelerate the healing process.

The application of hyssop oil to a wound creates an environment less favorable for bacterial growth, reducing the risk of infection. Furthermore, its anti-inflammatory properties may aid in reducing swelling and soothing the skin, fostering quicker recovery.

For bruises, hyssop may aid the healing process due to its potential to stimulate circulation. Increased blood flow to the affected area can expedite the healing of the bruise, reducing its visibility more quickly.

Hyssop's potential skin benefits extend beyond wound care. Some people use hyssop oil in skincare routines to help manage conditions like eczema or psoriasis, thanks to its potential anti-inflammatory and soothing properties. However, it's important to remember that essential oils, including hyssop, should always be diluted in a carrier oil before applying to the skin to prevent irritation.

Comfrey

Comfrey, also known as Symphytum officinale, has earned its nickname "knitbone" for a reason when it comes to healing soft tissue. With its large, hairy leaves and bell-shaped flowers, this plant is a true powerhouse for healing. One remarkable quality of comfrey is its high concentration of allantoin, a compound that stimulates the growth of new cells. This makes it an exceptional ally for bruises, sprains, and injuries, as it helps tissues come together and heal.

Comfrey shines in the plant kingdom for its ability to accelerate the healing process. Its potent combination of anti-inflammatory and pain-relieving properties can reduce swelling and pain while promoting the repair of damaged tissue. It works wonders for skin abrasions, minor burns, and even bone fractures, whether applied as a poultice, cream, or oil.

However, exercise CAUTION when using comfrey as it contains pyrrolizidine alkaloids, which can be harmful if ingested or excessively used on broken skin. Like any herbal remedy, responsible use and thorough research are essential.

Arnica

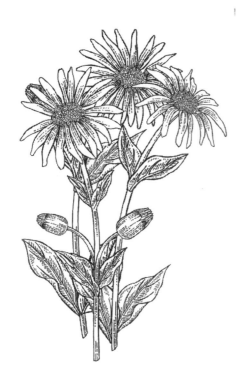

Arnica, specifically Arnica montana, is a vibrant yellow flower that grows in mountainous regions, and it's been used as a medicinal plant for centuries. It's a powerful healer that deserves a spot in your first-aid arsenal, especially regarding bruising and swelling.

The magic of arnica lies in its active compounds, like helenalin and dihydro helenalin, known for their anti-inflammatory and analgesic properties. When you apply arnica topically to a bruise, these compounds stimulate the activity of white blood cells that digest congested blood, thus reducing inflammation and swelling.

But that's not all. Arnica goes above and beyond. It has the power to alleviate trapped fluid in your joints, muscles, and bruised areas, giving your body a head start in the healing process and fading those bruises and discolorations faster.

One of the most common ways to use arnica is in the form of a gel or cream. Simply applying it to the affected area can significantly reduce healing time. Arnica-infused oils can also be used in a soothing massage to relieve muscle aches and pains.

Remember that arnica should only be used topically and for a short period. It can cause skin irritation in some people, especially with prolonged use. And it should never be applied to broken skin or open wounds due to the risk of absorption into the bloodstream.

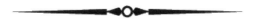

Recipes

Comfrey Poultice

Ingredients:

- Fresh comfrey leaves
- Water

Instructions:

1. Crush a handful of fresh comfrey leaves.

2. Add a little water to make a paste.

3. Spread the paste on a clean cloth and apply to the bruised area.

Prep Time: 10 minutes

Tips: Leave the poultice on for up to an hour. For sensitive skin, apply a thin layer of oil before using the poultice.

Plantain Infused Oil

Plantain has natural antibacterial and anti-inflammatory properties. It can be used to soothe and heal minor cuts and scrapes.

Ingredients:

- 1 cup fresh plantain leaves
- 2 cups of olive oil

Instructions:

1. Chop the plantain leaves and place them in a jar.

2. Pour the olive oil over the leaves until they are fully covered.

3. Place the jar in a sunny spot and let it infuse for 2-3 weeks.

4. Strain the oil into a clean jar.

Prep Time: 14-21 days

Tips: Use the oil as needed on cuts and scrapes. The oil can be stored in a cool, dark place for up to a year.

Yarrow Tea Rinse

Ingredients:

- 2 tablespoons of dried yarrow flowers
- 1 cup of boiling water

Instructions:

1. Place the yarrow flowers in a teapot or jar.

2. Pour the boiling water over the flowers.

3. Let the tea steep for at least 15 minutes.

4. Strain the tea and let it cool.

Prep Time: 20 minutes

Tips: Cleanse the wound with the cooled tea using a clean cloth or cotton ball. You can also use this as a compress on bruises to reduce swelling and discoloration.

Witch Hazel and Arnica Bruise Lotion

Ingredients:

- 1 cup of witch hazel

- 1 tablespoon of arnica flowers

- 1 tablespoon of aloe vera gel

- 1/4 cup of glycerin

Instructions:

1. Simmer the arnica flowers in the witch hazel in a double boiler for about 30 minutes.

2. Strain the mixture and allow it to cool.

3. Once cool, add the aloe vera gel and glycerin and stir until well mixed.

4. Store the lotion in a clean jar or bottle.

Prep Time: 1 hour

Tips: Apply the lotion gently on the bruised area two to three times daily. Do not apply on broken skin or open wounds. If any allergic reactions occur, discontinue use immediately.

Insect Bites and Stings

While most of these little nuisances only cause minor discomfort and itchiness, some can result in severe allergic reactions. Moreover, insects like mosquitoes can transmit diseases, making it even more important to tackle them promptly. But before you reach for synthetic creams or sprays, why not consider the power of nature?

Plantain

Plantain, scientifically known as Plantago major, may not be the most attractive plant, but it's exceptional at soothing insect bites and stings. It's a familiar sight in backyards and fields, often dismissed as a common weed. However, this underappreciated plant holds potent healing properties.

The plant's leaves contain anti-inflammatory substances as well as natural antihistamines. These properties make plantain an excellent choice for treating the itching and swelling caused by bug bites and stings. When applied, plantain goes to work, easing the itch and cooling the inflamed area, providing much-needed relief from the agony.

The extraordinary aspect of plantain lies not just in its effectiveness but also in its simplicity of use. You don't need any fancy concoctions to experience its benefits. Just find a leaf, give it a quick rinse, gently crush it between your fingers to release its healing juices, and apply it directly to the affected area. The relief is often immediate and remarkable, showing the actual potency of plantain.

Basil

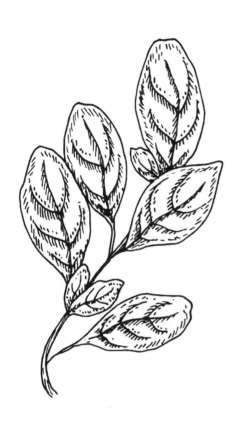

Basil (Ocimum basilicum), a beloved herb found in many kitchens, not only adds a delightful aroma to our culinary creations but also offers valuable properties for soothing and healing. Its distinct fragrance, a delightful blend of sweet and herbal notes, is instantly recognizable and evokes a sense of familiarity in our kitchens.

This herb is rich in volatile oils such as camphor and thymol, which provide a cooling sensation that can help alleviate itching and inflammation. Basil (Ocimum basilicum) also possesses antimicrobial properties, which may help prevent infection, a potential concern, especially with insect bites that have been scratched.

Basil can be used in multiple ways to help with insect bites. For instance, you can crush fresh basil leaves to release the beneficial oils, then apply the mashed leaves directly to the bite for immediate relief. The cooling sensation can soothe the affected area and reduce the urge to scratch.

For a refreshing and easy-to-make solution, try basil-infused water that can be used as a spray for insect bites. Begin by gathering a handful of fresh basil leaves and steeping them in hot water for approximately 20 minutes. This allows the water to extract the beneficial compounds from the basil. Once the water has cooled, transfer it to a spray bottle or use a cotton ball to dab the infused water onto the affected area. Feel free to reapply as needed for soothing relief. The combination of the basil's properties and the coolness of the water can provide a refreshing and comforting sensation, helping to alleviate the discomfort caused by insect bites.

Witch Hazel

Witch Hazel, or Hamamelis virginiana, is an unassuming shrub native to North America that has been championed in folk medicine for generations. Its unique astringent and anti-inflammatory properties make it an excellent ally against insect bites and stings.

The power of witch hazel lies in its ability to soothe and reduce swelling, while its astringent properties help to tighten the skin and relieve itching. It's like a mini, natural first-aid kit packed into a single plant.

Typically, witch hazel is used as a distilled extract, which concentrates its healing properties. Often found in health stores or online, this extract can be applied directly to the insect bite or sting. You'll feel the cooling, soothing sensation almost immediately as the witch hazel goes to work, reducing inflammation and easing the relentless itch that often accompanies insect bites.

What makes witch hazel even more appealing is its versatility. It's not just limited to insect bites and stings. The same properties that make it effective for these uses also make it an excellent choice for many other skin issues, including acne, eczema, and even hemorrhoids.

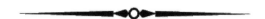

Recipes

<u>Witch Hazel Spray</u>

Witch hazel is well-known for its astringent and anti-inflammatory properties, helping to reduce swelling and calm irritation.

- *Ingredients*
  - 1/2 cup witch hazel extract
  - 1/2 cup distilled water
  - 10 drops of tea tree essential oil
- *Instructions*
  - Mix witch hazel extract, water, and tea tree essential oil in a spray bottle.
  - Shake well before each use.
  - Spray onto the affected area as needed.
- *Prep time*: 10 minutes
- *Tips*: Always test a small area of skin first to ensure there's no adverse reaction to the solution.

<u>Lavender Essential Oil</u>

Lavender is prized for its soothing properties and ability to promote healing and reduce inflammation.

- *Ingredients*
  - Lavender essential oil
  - A carrier oil (like coconut or jojoba oil)
- *Instructions*
  - Mix a few drops of lavender essential oil with a teaspoon of carrier oil.
  - Apply the mixture to the affected area for relief.
- *Prep time*: 5 minutes
- *Tips*: Essential oils are potent; always dilute them with a carrier oil before applying to the skin.

<u>Chamomile Tea Compress</u>

Chamomile is used for its calming and anti-inflammatory properties, reducing redness and swelling.

- *Ingredients*
  - 1 chamomile tea bag
  - Hot water
- *Instructions*
  - Steep the chamomile tea bag in hot water for 5-10 minutes.
  - Let the tea cool to a comfortable temperature.
  - Soak a clean cloth in the tea, and wring out the excess liquid.
  - Apply the cloth to the affected area as a compress.
  - Leave on for 15-20 minutes.

Prep time: 15 minutes

Tips: You can also use chamomile essential oil mixed with a carrier oil for similar effects.

Chapter Two

Herbal First Aid - Part II

Poison Ivy and Other Skin Irritants

Coming into contact with poison ivy or other skin irritants can quickly turn a lovely day outdoors into a week-long itching and discomfort. The urushiol oil in poison ivy causes a rash ranging from mildly annoying to extremely painful. Don't despair, though - nature's apothecary has a few herbal remedies that can help to soothe and heal your irritated skin. Let's dive in and explore some of the most effective ones.

St. John's Wort

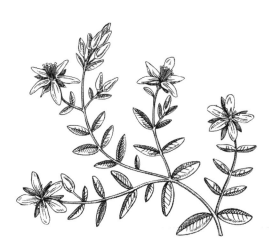

St. John's Wort, also known as Hypericum perforatum, is more than just a mood enhancer. This herb is a powerful remedy for relieving skin irritations like poison ivy. Packed with active compounds like hypericin and hyperforin, it offers anti-inflammatory, antimicrobial, and pain-relieving effects. Applied topically as an oil, cream, or salve, St. John's Wort soothes discomfort and reduces inflammation caused by poison ivy and similar irritants.

The alleviating action of St. John's Wort on troubled skin stems from its ability to reduce redness, swelling, and itching, thanks to its anti-inflammatory nature. Additionally, its antimicrobial qualities help ward off potential secondary infections that can crop up when irritants compromise the skin's protective barrier. Plus, it can ease the pain often associated with skin irritations, courtesy of its analgesic properties.

For optimal results against poison ivy and other skin irritants, it is recommended to use a topical application of St. John's Wort-infused oil, cream, or salve. This can provide soothing relief and promote healing. Apply directly to the affected area multiple times daily to ease the skin, diminish inflammation, and support healing. Bear in mind that St. John's Wort can make your skin more sensitive to the sun, so avoiding direct sunlight or protecting the treated area is necessary.

Jewelweed

Jewelweed (Impatiens capensis), with its distinctive orange or yellow flowers, has been a trusted ally in the plant world for generations, especially when dealing with skin irritants like poison ivy. This humble plant, also known as Impatiens capensis, is much more than just a pretty face. Commonly found in the same environment as poison ivy, it's as if nature purposely placed the antidote next to it.

The power of jewelweed can be found in its succulent stems and leaves, which are filled with translucent juice. When applied to the skin, this juice works wonders. It helps to counteract the urushiol oil from poison ivy that causes all the itching and discomfort. The compounds in jewelweed can bind with urushiol oil, neutralizing its irritating effects and preventing it from spreading.

To use jewelweed, break open the stem or a leaf and apply the juice directly to your skin. Doing this as soon as possible after coming into contact with poison ivy is crucial to prevent the urushiol oil from fully bonding with your skin. Ideally, you'd want to have jewelweed on hand during any outdoor activity where you might encounter poison ivy.

Jewelweed can also be made into a bar of soap or a salve that can be stored for extended periods. You can prepare it in advance and keep it in your first aid kit. This way, you'll have the remedy ready, even if there's no fresh jewelweed around when needed.

Oatmeal

Oatmeal, a modest pantry staple, has an unexpected role in skin care, particularly when dealing with skin irritants like poison ivy. This common grain may not be considered a 'herb,' but its tremendous calming effects make it an essential member of this list.

Oatmeal is packed with avenanthramides, known for their anti-inflammatory and antioxidant properties. When applied topically, these compounds help to reduce itching, inflammation, and redness associated with poison ivy. They work by calming the skin, reducing inflammation, and forming a protective layer over the skin that helps to retain its natural moisture, speeding up the healing process.

The most frequent and effective way to reap the advantages of oats is to take an oatmeal bath. It's an easy, soothing, and time-tested treatment. To make an oatmeal bath, grind one cup of raw, whole oats in a blender or food processor until they form a fine powder colloquially known as "colloidal oatmeal." Fill your bathtub with lukewarm water, and while the tub is filling, slowly sprinkle the ground oatmeal into the tub, stirring the water with your hand to help disperse the oatmeal. Soak in the oatmeal bath for about 15 to 20 minutes. After the bath, lightly rinse your body with lukewarm water without using soap and pat your skin dry.

An oatmeal bath not only helps to soothe the irritation caused by poison ivy but also provides an overall calming effect that can be especially beneficial if your sleep has been disrupted due to itching.

Tips: Remember to exercise caution when using oatmeal for poison ivy treatment. While oatmeal baths are generally safe and well-tolerated, some individuals may be allergic or sensitive to oats. It is recommended to perform a patch test before using oatmeal topically to ensure there are no adverse reactions. Additionally, if symptoms worsen or persist, seek medical attention.

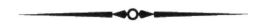

While we've already discussed the excellent properties of Calendula, Plantain, and Aloe Vera, it's worth mentioning them again when it comes to addressing skin irritation. These herbs have proven effective in providing relief and promoting skin healing. These three are a dynamic trio in the herbal world, each bringing unique capabilities. Calendula, a champion of wound healing, has anti-inflammatory effects. Plantain is excellent in drawing out poisons, making it a must-have for insect bites or poison ivy reactions. Then there's Aloe Vera, well-known for its soothing and cooling properties, providing quick relief from burns and rashes. They create a fantastic team capable of combating many skin irritations.

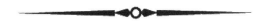

Recipes

Plantain Salve

Plantain (Plantago major) is a ubiquitous plant that grows in yards, parks, and wild places. It has astringent properties that draw out toxins and anti-inflammatory properties that reduce swelling and itching. This salve can be applied directly to skin irritated by poison ivy.

Ingredients:

- 1 cup fresh plantain leaves
- 1 cup olive oil
- 1/4 cup beeswax pellets
- Small glass jar

Instructions:

1. Wash and dry the plantain leaves.
2. Chop the leaves finely and put them in a glass jar.
3. Pour the olive oil into the jar, making sure to completely cover the leaves.
4. Put the jar in a slow cooker filled with a few inches of water and let it infuse on the low setting for about 8 hours.
5. Strain the oil, discard the leaves, and return the oil to the cleaned jar.
6. Melt the beeswax in a double boiler, then mix it into the oil, stirring until well combined.
7. Let the salve cool before putting the lid on the jar.

Prep Time: 9 hours

Tip: Keep the salve in a cool, dry place and use it within a year.

Jewelweed Lotion

Ingredients:

- 2 cups fresh jewelweed stems and leaves

- 1 cup coconut oil

- 1/2 cup aloe vera gel

- Essential oils (optional)

Instructions:

1. Rinse and chop the jewelweed.

2. Put the jewelweed, coconut oil, and aloe vera gel into a blender or food processor.

3. Blend until smooth.

4. Strain the mixture through a fine mesh strainer or cheesecloth.

5. Add a few drops of essential oil for fragrance, if desired.

6. Store in a small glass jar.

Prep Time: 30 minutes

Tip: Dried jewelweed can be used if you don't have fresh jewelweed, but note that the fresh plant is more potent.

Calendula and Lavender Bath Soak

Ingredients:

- 1 cup dried calendula flowers

- 1/2 cup dried lavender flowers

- 1 cup Epsom salts

- Muslin bag

Instructions:

1. Mix the calendula flowers, lavender flowers, and Epsom salts in a bowl.

2. Put the mixture in a muslin bag.

3. Draw a warm bath and add the muslin bag to the water.

4. Soak in the bath for 20-30 minutes.

Prep Time: 5 minutes (not including bath time)

Tip: This mixture can also be used as a foot soak. Add a few drops of lavender essential oil to the bathwater for an extra soothing touch.

Witch Hazel and Aloe Spray

Ingredients:

- 1/2 cup witch hazel

- 1/2 cup aloe vera gel

- 10 drops of lavender essential oil

- 10 drops of tea tree essential oil

Instructions:

1. Combine the witch hazel and aloe vera gel in a bowl.

2. Add the essential oils and stir well to combine.

3. Pour the mixture into a spray bottle.

4. Shake well before each use and spray liberally onto affected areas.

Prep Time: 5 minutes

Tip: Store the spray in the refrigerator for an extra cooling effect when applied. The aloe vera in this recipe is soothing and moisturizing, helping to heal the skin.

Toothaches and Gum Issues

Toothaches and gum problems can be highly annoying, interfering with our daily lives with constant discomfort or pain. While it is always necessary to consult a dentist for recurring issues, several herbal therapies can provide relief while supporting overall oral health.

Clove

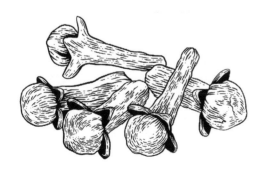

Clove (Syzygium aromaticum) has a rich history of use for medicinal purposes, dating back to ancient civilizations. The Chinese have used clove for over 2,000 years to treat various ailments, including toothaches and digestive issues. This versatile spice has also been used in traditional Indian Ayurvedic medicine for its numerous health benefits.

When dealing with tooth issues, the active ingredient in clove, eugenol, is a natural solution. This powerful compound offers multiple benefits for dental health. For instance, it alleviates pain by numbing the affected area, bringing much-needed relief to those suffering from toothaches. Also, eugenol's antibacterial properties combat the bacteria that may be causing or exacerbating dental problems, such as tooth decay or gum disease.

There are different ways to use clove for dental health:

- Clove Oil: check the recipe in the following section

- Whole Clove: Gently chew an entire clove to release the oil and benefit from its pain-relieving and antibacterial properties.

Myrrh

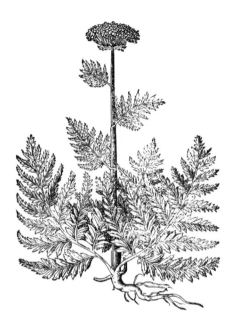

The intriguing resin of the myrrh tree, known scientifically as Commiphora myrrha, has been an esteemed natural remedy dating back to ancient times. With astringent and antimicrobial properties, myrrh stands out as a valuable resource for oral health. Notably, it helps firm up the gums and fight against harmful bacteria, which can lead to various dental issues.

Myrrh, which is a lesser-known gem in the world of herbal remedies, was once so valued that it was used as a currency in ancient Egypt. Moreover, it was among the gifts the three wise men brought to the baby Jesus in the biblical account.

Now, to prepare a homemade myrrh mouthwash, the steps are simple. Start by placing a teaspoon of myrrh powder into 2 cups of water. Allow it to simmer gently for about 30 minutes. Once it has sufficiently cooled, you can use it as a rinse for your mouth multiple times daily. This humble, DIY remedy can be a game-changer in maintaining your oral health while connecting you to an ancient tradition of natural healing.

Neem

Neem (Azadirachta indica), often called the "pharmacy tree," has numerous medicinal properties that have been utilized for thousands of years in Ayurvedic medicine.

Neem offers several advantages for maintaining healthy teeth and gums:

Antibacterial Properties - Neem's antibacterial properties help to combat the bacteria that cause tooth decay and gum disease.

Anti-inflammatory Properties – Neem can reduce inflammation in the gums, alleviating discomfort and improving overall gum health.

Natural Solution – As a natural remedy, neem provides a gentle alternative to harsh chemical treatments for oral health issues.

There are various ways to incorporate neem into your oral care routine:

- Neem Leaves: Chewing on neem leaves can help maintain overall dental health by using the plant's antibacterial and anti-inflammatory qualities.

- Neem Oil: Applying neem oil to the gums can reduce inflammation and combat bacteria, promoting healthy gum tissue.

Neem's remarkable healing properties have earned it the nickname "village pharmacy" in India. In addition to its benefits for oral health, neem has been used traditionally to treat a wide range of ailments, including skin conditions, digestive issues, and even malaria.

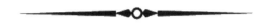

Recipes

Clove Oil Toothache Drop

Ingredients:

- 1 tablespoon of Olive Oil

- 5-7 Clove Buds

Instructions:

1. Crush the clove buds into a fine powder.

2. Mix the powder with the olive oil.

3. Apply a drop to the painful area using a cotton swab.

Prep Time: 10 minutes

Tip: Always apply the clove oil mixture with a cotton swab to avoid irritating other areas of the mouth.

Sage Mouth Rinse

Sage is a potent antimicrobial herb that has been used for centuries for dental hygiene. It can alleviate sore gums and cleanse the oral cavity, promoting overall dental health.

Ingredients:

- 1 cup of Water

- 2 tablespoons of Dried Sage

Instructions:

- Boil the water.

- Add the dried sage and simmer for 10 minutes.

- Let it cool down, then use it as a mouth rinse, swishing it for 1 minute.

Prep Time: 20 minutes

Tip: This rinse can be made in larger batches and stored in the refrigerator for up to a week.

Thyme Essential Oil Toothpaste

Thyme is recognized for its potent antibacterial and antifungal properties, making it excellent for preventing tooth decay and gum disease.

Ingredients:

- 2 tablespoons of Coconut Oil
- 2 tablespoons of Baking Soda
- 10 drops of Thyme Essential Oil

Instructions:

1. Melt the coconut oil in a small bowl.
2. Mix in the baking soda to form a paste.
3. Add the thyme essential oil and mix well.
4. Use as you would regular toothpaste.

Prep Time: 10 minutes

Tips: It's best to use this toothpaste sparingly, as essential oils can be quite strong. You can make small batches and keep them in a cool, dry place to maintain their freshness.

Turmeric Gum Paste

Ingredients:

- 1 teaspoon of Turmeric Powder
- A small amount of Water

Instructions:

- Mix turmeric powder with just enough water to form a thick paste.
- Apply this paste to the gums and let it sit for 5 minutes.
- Rinse thoroughly with warm water.

Prep Time: 5 minutes

Tip: To avoid staining, rinse your mouth thoroughly after using turmeric paste.

Peppermint Tea Mouthwash

Everyone knows peppermint for its refreshing aroma and cooling effects. But did you know that it contains antibacterial properties, which can help fight oral pathogens? That's right; Peppermint's antibacterial properties help to inhibit the growth of harmful bacteria in the mouth, reducing the risk of dental issues and promoting a healthier oral environment.

Ingredients:

- 1 Peppermint Tea Bag

- 1 cup of Boiling Water

Instructions:

1. Steep the peppermint tea bag in boiling water for 10 minutes.

2. Allow it to cool, then use it as a mouthwash. Swish it in your mouth for 1 minute and then spit it out.

Prep Time: 15 minutes

Tips: This mouthwash can be used twice daily, in the morning and before bed, for a refreshing breath. Avoid swallowing the mouthwash.

BOOK V

HERBAL BEAUTY AND SKINCARE

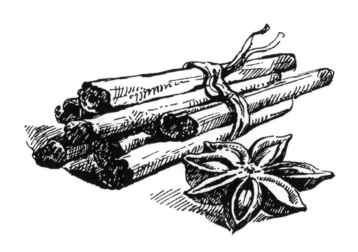

AMBER WHITMORE

Introduction

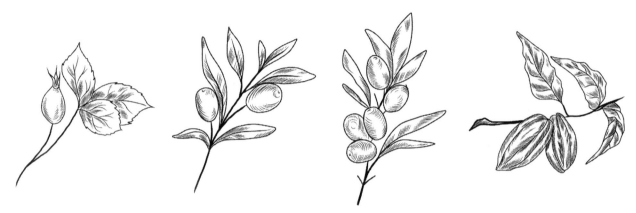

For millennia, natural remedies have been the foundation of skincare routines. Evidence demonstrates that ancient civilizations, such as the Egyptians and Greeks, had their own distinctive mixtures of natural elements that were deemed to enhance visual appeal. Aloe Vera, olive oil, and other botanicals were widely employed, each picked for its supposed beneficial virtues. These methods, which have been passed down through centuries, have created a rich skincare heritage based on the treasures of the natural world.

In our modern era, marked by the rise of technology and synthetic substances, there appears to be an inclination toward these traditional natural practices. The drive to adopt more natural and sustainable lifestyles has brought herbal remedies into the spotlight, which is reflected in the beauty industry, where 'green' or 'natural' products are increasingly sought after, and artificial substances, like parabens and sulfates, are being shunned.

In the following pages, we'll uncover the world of herbal beauty and skincare, various essential herbs, their specific benefits for the skin, and how they can be used to address everyday skincare concerns. Also, we'll discuss how to incorporate these herbal remedies into daily skincare routines, even offering guidance on making your herbal products at home.

Chapter One
Understanding Skin Biology

Beneath the touch of your fingertips, under the mirror's gaze, is an incredibly complex and fascinating organ – the skin. This vital frontier guards us from the outside world while simultaneously presenting ourselves to it.

Skin Structure

Imagine the skin as a multilayered cake. The topmost layer, the one that meets the eye and the world, is the epidermis. Mainly consisting of cells known as keratinocytes, the epidermis is our protective shield. It's continually regenerating, with new cells pushing their way up from the bottom, hardening and packing tightly together as they rise. By the time they reach the surface, they are dead, flat, and ready to flake off - creating space for a fresh battalion. This natural process is our body's brilliant strategy for protecting us from environmental aggressors.

But the epidermis is not just about defense. Its lower regions are home to the melanocytes, the cells responsible for the pigment in our skin, hair, and eyes. The diversity of human skin tones, from the palest white to the deepest brown, is the handiwork of these very cells and their pigment production, also known as melanin.

Beneath the epidermis lies the dermis, the second layer of the skin, the structural layer. Imagine this as the supportive mattress of the skin cake, sturdier and thicker than the topmost layer. This layer is bustling with collagen and elastin, two protein types that give skin strength, flexibility, and resilience. The dermis also hosts a myriad of blood vessels, sweat glands, hair follicles, and nerve endings.

The deepest layer of our skin is the subcutaneous layer or hypodermis, composed mainly of fat cells. This layer acts as a shock absorber, conserves body heat, and provides nutritional support to the other skin layers.

The architecture of our skin is continually adapting to internal and external factors. It's an impressive organ, constantly working, endlessly renewing, and subtly communicating with the rest of the body. As we unravel the language of our skin and understand its structure, we're better equipped to care for it and appreciate its needs. Taking a holistic approach to skincare allows us to appreciate the beauty of our skin, not just in its appearance but also in its function and overall health.

Functions of the skin

More than just a cover, our skin works tirelessly around the clock, conducting a symphony of tasks that keep us healthy and protected.

The most prominent role of our skin is to act as a barrier. Just like a dedicated security guard, the skin stands at the front line, defending our bodies against various external threats. These include harmful microorganisms, toxins, and damaging UV rays from the sun. Consider a day at the beach. Our skin bears the brunt of the intense sun, with its upper layer - the epidermis - producing extra melanin to shield the deeper cells from harmful radiation.

In addition, the skin functions as a sentinel for our sense of touch. The dermis layer's massive network of nerves communicates with our brain, allowing us to feel tactile sensations. Think about the last time you held a soft kitten, felt the prickle of a thorny rose, or felt the warmth of a loved one's hand in yours. We can perceive these many feelings because of these nerve endings.

Our skin also plays a vital role in body temperature regulation. It does so through thermoregulation, managed by sweat glands and blood vessels housed in the dermis. When we're overheated, perhaps from a strenuous workout, our skin sweats, releasing warmth and cooling us down. In contrast, when we're cold, the blood vessels in the skin constrict, preserving body heat.

Additionally, the skin actively participates in our body's immune response. Specialized cells in the epidermis, called Langerhans cells, are constantly looking for pathogens. When they spot trouble, they alert the immune system to spring into action, warding off potential infections.

Our skin is a silent partner in the body's vitamin D production, a nutrient crucial for bone health. When UVB rays from the sun hit the skin, a series of biochemical reactions get triggered, leading to the synthesis of Vitamin D. So, while we all enjoy the warmth of the sun, it's comforting to know that our skin is also benefiting from it. Remember that it's crucial to protect our skin from its potential harm. Incorporating sunscreen creams into our skincare routine is essential to prevent sunburn, premature aging, and damage caused by harmful UVA and UVB rays.

How to Keep Your Skin Healthy

Understanding our skin's complex structure and functions is fundamental in adopting a holistic approach to skincare. However, knowing is only half the battle. The next step is to translate this understanding into action and establish habits that support and nourish our skin. Here are some natural strategies you can incorporate into your lifestyle to keep your skin healthy and radiant:

1. Nourish from Within

Remember the saying, "You are what you eat?" This adage rings particularly true for skin health. The foods you consume can significantly affect the health and aging of your skin. For a glowing complexion, incorporate a diet rich in fruits, vegetables, lean proteins, and healthy fats. These foods are packed with vitamins, antioxidants, and omega-3 fatty acids, which promote skin health.

For instance, consider adding berries to your morning cereal or yogurt. Berries are rich in antioxidants, which protect your skin from the damaging effects of free radicals. Similarly, avocados are high in healthy fats and vitamins E and C, known for their skin-enhancing properties.

2. Stay Hydrated

The essence of healthy skin is hydration. Drinking plenty of water maintains skin elasticity and suppleness. Additionally, it aids in flushing out toxins, keeping your skin clear and radiant. Remember, when we're well-hydrated, our skin cells function at their best. So, always keep a reusable water bottle with you as a friendly reminder to drink up!

3. Prioritize Sleep

Sleep is when your body, including your skin, goes into repair mode. Lack of adequate sleep can result in dark circles, dull skin, and even breakouts. Establish a regular sleep schedule and aim for seven to nine hours of quality sleep each night. Consider this your beauty sleep.

4. Avoid Sun Damage

While sun exposure is essential for vitamin D production, too much sun can cause skin damage, including wrinkles and an increased risk of skin cancer. So, apply a broad-spectrum sunscreen with SPF 30 or higher whenever you're stepping out, even on cloudy days.

5. Practice Gentle Skin Care

Regarding skincare routines, remember the principle of 'less is more.' Overwashing or excessive exfoliation can strip your skin of its natural oils, leading to dryness and irritation. Opt for gentle, natural products, and remember to moisturize daily. Treat your skin like delicate fabric - it requires a gentle touch.

Consider, for instance, the traditional practice of oil cleansing, where plant-based oils are used to remove makeup and impurities. This practice not only cleanses but also hydrates and balances the skin.

6. Manage Stress

High-stress levels can trigger skin issues like breakouts and other skin problems. Various techniques like yoga, meditation, and deep breathing can help manage stress levels and promote skin health and overall well-being.

Remember, skin health is not just about appearance; it indicates your body's overall health. Listen to your skin and care for it with the love and respect it deserves. Following these guidelines lets you maintain your skin's health naturally and beautifully.

Chapter Two
Herbal Remedies for Common Skin Concerns

Acne

Let's explore some herbal superheroes and see how they can help your skin against acne.

Green Tea

Green tea is not just a flavorful beverage but also provides numerous skincare benefits. Rich in antioxidants and tannins, green tea helps regulate sebum production, which is a significant factor in the development of acne. By acting as a moderator, green tea effectively manages the oil flow on the skin, preventing clogged pores and the subsequent formation of acne.

Witch Hazel

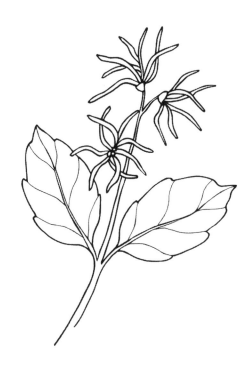

Witch hazel, scientifically known as Hamamelis virginiana, is a plant native to North America. This small tree or shrub is well-regarded in traditional medicine for its unique healing properties, mainly derived from its leaves and bark. Often distilled into a liquid extract or included in various skincare products, witch hazel has become a staple in natural wellness and skincare regimens around the world.

One of the most common and well-researched uses of witch hazel is its application in treating acne. This skin condition, characterized by inflamed, often painful skin lesions, can occur at any age, though it's most prevalent among teenagers. The search for effective, affordable, and easy-to-use remedies has led many to explore herbal options, with witch hazel standing out as a prime candidate.

Witch hazel contains tannins, a type of natural compound with potent antioxidant and astringent properties. When applied to the skin, witch hazel can help to reduce excess oil production, one of the leading contributors to the formation of acne. By reducing oil (sebum) and tightening the skin, it helps to create an inhospitable environment for the bacteria that exacerbate acne.

In addition to regulating oil production, witch hazel's anti-inflammatory properties can help to reduce the redness and swelling associated with acne. This makes it a two-fold treatment, addressing both the cause and the visible symptoms of acne.

Using witch hazel as an acne treatment typically involves applying a small amount of witch hazel extract to a clean cotton ball or pad and gently dabbing it onto the affected area. For optimal results, this can be incorporated into daily skincare routines, typically after cleansing and before moisturizing.

Furthermore, witch hazel's skin-soothing properties can help to calm irritation that often accompanies frequent acne breakouts, and its gentle nature makes it suitable for most skin types.

Turmeric

This radiant golden spice brings more to the table than color and flavor. Turmeric, particularly the active ingredient curcumin, has powerful anti-inflammatory and antibacterial benefits. These properties can reduce the inflammation surrounding acne, and their antibacterial action aids in tackling the bacteria contributing to acne's development. Thus, turmeric can be considered a two-pronged warrior, combating acne on multiple fronts.

Tea Tree Oil

Tea tree oil can be particularly beneficial for various forms of skin damage. Whether the issue is acne, psoriasis, or cuts and scrapes, this essential oil has proven a remarkably effective herbal remedy.

Acne - Due to its antibacterial properties, tea tree oil is commonly used to treat acne. Applying it topically (in diluted form) helps reduce inflammation and kill bacteria that can lead to breakouts. Some studies have even found tea tree oil to be as effective as benzoyl peroxide, a common ingredient in acne treatments, but without harsh side effects such as skin irritation and dryness.

Wound Healing - Tea tree oil can promote wound healing due to its antiseptic properties, which prevent infections, and anti-inflammatory properties, which reduce inflammation. When used correctly, it can expedite the healing process of minor cuts, scrapes, and insect bites.

Psoriasis and Eczema - These skin conditions can cause inflammation, itching, and discomfort. With its anti-inflammatory and soothing properties, tea tree oil can alleviate symptoms and reduce flare-ups. However, it's important to note that tea tree oil can help manage symptoms but doesn't cure these conditions.

Fungal Infections - Tea tree oil is known for its antifungal abilities, making it helpful in treating conditions like athlete's foot or nail fungus.

When using tea tree oil, it's crucial to remember that it should never be ingested and always be diluted before being applied to the skin. Moreover, some individuals may be allergic to tea tree oil, so a patch test should be performed before full application.

Skin Dryness

Here, we spotlight five plant-based remedies that stand out in their abilities to quench the skin's thirst.

Chamomile

Recognized and loved for its calming effects when sipped as a tea, chamomile also offers soothing, anti-inflammatory properties for the skin. Used as a tea rinse or an infused oil, this daisy-like plant comforts dry, inflamed skin with its healing touch. Chamomile also contains flavonoids and antioxidants that can penetrate below the skin's surface. Chamomile is like a gentle friend offering a soft, comforting blanket, draping your skin with hydration while soothing any irritation that often accompanies dryness.

Olive Oil

Olive oil, a staple in Mediterranean cuisine, is an excellent hydrator for dehydrated skin. Rich in beneficial monounsaturated fats and vitamin E, olive oil nourishes the skin deeply, combating dryness and enhancing skin elasticity. When applied topically, envision it as a nurturing protector, fortifying your skin's natural barrier, locking in moisture, and warding off environmental stressors that can exacerbate dryness.

Jojoba Oil

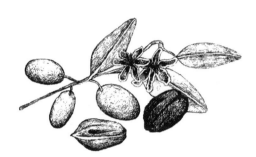

Harvested from the seeds of the desert-dwelling Simmondsia chinensis plant, jojoba oil is a natural skincare marvel. Its unique structure closely mirrors our skin's sebum, enabling it to moisturize without tipping the scales toward oiliness. Moreover, jojoba oil creates a soft, protective layer on your skin, preventing moisture loss through evaporation. Jojoba oil can be your skin's trusty backup, ready to replenish moisture reserves whenever levels dip too low.

Honey

Honey, nature's sweet gift, is a fantastic moisturizer that has stood the test of time in skincare. Its humectant properties attract moisture, while its rich antioxidants, enzymes, and nutrients nourish the skin. Honey is also known for its gentle exfoliating properties, helping remove dead skin cells that often give dry skin a dull appearance. Consider honey as your skincare artisan, skillfully attracting, sealing, and preserving moisture while gently polishing your skin for a radiant glow.

Aging Skin / Wrinkles

As we all know, aging is a natural process, and the appearance of wrinkles is a testament to a life well-lived. Yet, it's completely natural to wish for a youthful glow. Fortunately, herbal remedies offer a gentle, natural approach to skin care for aging skin and wrinkles.

Rosehip Oil

Derived from the tiny, nutrient-packed seeds of wild rose bushes, rosehip oil boasts a wealth of skin-nourishing elements. Packed with vitamins A and C and essential fatty acids, it promotes skin regeneration, boosts collagen production, and provides hydration for a youthful and plump complexion. With its skin-renewing properties, rosehip oil works wonders in reducing the appearance of wrinkles and fine lines, giving your skin a healthy and radiant glow.

Pomegranate

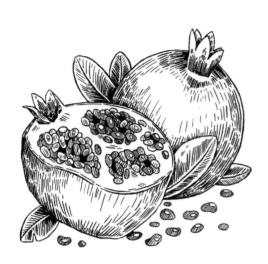

Pomegranate, botanically known as Punica granatum, is a versatile and potent medicinal plant known across various cultures for its array of health benefits. Bearing ruby-red seeds, or arils, nestled within its round, leathery skin, this 'jewel of the winter' is more than just a delightful, juicy fruit. It holds a coveted place in the realm of herbal remedies, particularly for its benefits to the skin, especially aging skin.

Aging skin, characterized by wrinkles, fine lines, and age spots, is primarily the result of oxidative stress, leading to damage at the cellular level. Pomegranates are packed with antioxidants, including polyphenols and vitamin C, which help counteract this oxidative stress. They neutralize harmful free radicals in the body, reducing cellular damage and slowing the aging process.

Promoting Collagen Production

Collagen is a vital protein that keeps the skin firm and youthful. As we age, collagen production decreases, leading to wrinkles and sagging skin. Pomegranates contain compounds that protect the breakdown of collagen and may boost its production, thus helping to maintain skin elasticity and reduce the appearance of wrinkles.

Deep Hydration and Skin Repair

Pomegranate seed oil, extracted from the arils, is a rich source of punicic acid, an omega-5 fatty acid known for its powerful hydrating properties. It penetrates deep into the skin, providing intense moisture and nourishment. This aids in skin repair and rejuvenation, further helping in the reduction of wrinkles and fine lines.

Enhanced Sun Protection

Another important aspect of aging skin is the increased vulnerability to sun damage. Pomegranate offers a measure of photoprotection. Its antioxidants reduce the damage caused by harmful UV rays, preventing premature aging of the skin.

Incorporating Pomegranate into Your Skin Care Routine

Incorporating pomegranate into your skincare routine can be as simple as consuming the fresh fruit or its juice for internal benefits. For external application, consider pomegranate-infused skincare products like creams, serums, or oils. Alternatively, pomegranate seed oil can be directly applied to the skin.

Frankincense

This fragrant resin, which has been treasured since ancient times, gives us its skin rejuvenating properties. As a natural astringent, frankincense can tighten the skin, reducing the appearance of pores and wrinkles. Used frequently in oils or creams, this botanical wonder can refine and reshape your skin's texture and appearance, imparting a youthful glow.

Licorice Root

Licorice root is no ordinary herb. It contains powerful compounds like glycyrrhizin acid and liquiritin that work wonders for your skin health. These exhibit skin-brightening properties, improve skin elasticity, and diminish the appearance of wrinkles and age spots.

Sensitive Skin and Inflammation

Maintaining the health of sensitive skin also demands attention to lifestyle choices, including a balanced diet, adequate hydration, and stress management. Some botanical solutions can relieve and manage sensitive skin and inflammation.

Calendula

Derived from marigold flowers, calendula is appreciated for its calming and healing properties. Its potent anti-inflammatory, antifungal, and antibacterial properties help soothe the skin, reduce redness, and speed up the healing of any minor skin irritations. Calendula is a gentle healer that can provide immediate comfort and promote quick recovery for distressed skin.

Oatmeal

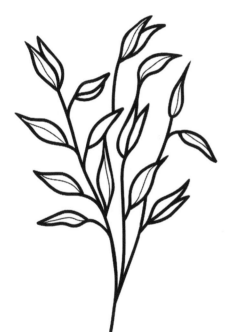

When we think of oatmeal, breakfast likely comes to mind. However, this versatile grain, known scientifically as Avena sativa, extends its benefits beyond the breakfast bowl. Traditional herbal medicine has recognized the potential of oatmeal as a health remedy for centuries, particularly in skin care and inflammation management.

Oatmeal for Sensitive Skin

Oatmeal is a renowned ally for sensitive skin. It's packed with compounds like avenanthramides, which have been found to exhibit anti-inflammatory and anti-itch properties. A warm, soothing oatmeal bath is a traditional home remedy for many skin issues, ranging from dry, itchy skin to more severe conditions like eczema and psoriasis. The grains' gentle exfoliating properties can also help remove dead skin cells, leaving the skin softer and smoother.

For a simple oatmeal skin treatment, finely ground oats can be mixed with warm water to form a paste, which can then be applied to the affected area. Alternatively, whole oats can be added to bathwater for a full-body soak. The resulting milky bathwater offers a calming, soothing treatment for irritated skin.

Oatmeal for Inflammation

In addition to relieving sensitive skin, oatmeal has potential benefits in managing inflammation. The avenanthramides in oats have strong antioxidant properties, which help fight off the damaging effects of inflammation. They can help the body manage inflammatory conditions and potentially prevent chronic diseases associated with oxidative stress.

A diet rich in oats can provide these benefits internally, but oatmeal can also be used topically to manage localized inflammation. An oatmeal poultice – a cloth filled with cooked, cooled oatmeal – can be applied directly to inflamed areas to soothe and reduce swelling.

Chamomile

A familiar name in skincare, chamomile, be it in the form of tea, oil, or infused in creams, is a true friend of sensitive skin. Its antioxidant and anti-inflammatory compounds can help alleviate skin irritations, redness, and itchiness. Chamomile is a soothing herb, always ready to calm and comfort your troubled skin.

Lavender

Renowned for its enchanting aroma, lavender, in oil form or skin care products, offers many benefits for sensitive skin. Its anti-inflammatory and antiseptic properties can help relieve inflammation and prevent infections. I would say lavender is a gentle whisperer, calming the uproars of inflammation and guarding against potential intruders.

Skin Damages

Our skin often falls prey to damage from sun exposure and scarring. Here are some herbal remedies that are well-equipped to repair damaged skin.

St. John's Wort

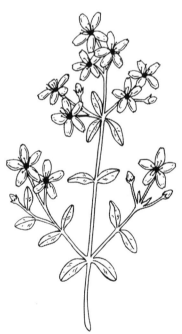

St. John's Wort, known scientifically as Hypericum perforatum, is a flowering plant native to parts of Europe and Asia but can also be found in temperate regions worldwide. This herb, easily recognizable by its bright yellow flowers, has been a staple in traditional medicine for centuries. Although it is often associated with mental health and has been widely studied for its potential benefits in managing depression, St. John's Wort also offers impressive benefits for skin health.

<u>Healing Power on Skin Damages</u>

St. John's Wort has been celebrated for its anti-inflammatory, antibacterial, and astringent properties, contributing to its reputation as a potent remedy for various skin conditions. The herb's skin-friendly properties are mainly attributed to hyperforin and hypericin, compounds known to accelerate wound healing and skin repair.

Wound Healing – St. John's Wort can be applied topically to wounds, cuts, burns, and abrasions to promote healing. Its natural antibacterial properties protect the wound from infection, while its anti-inflammatory effects help reduce swelling and inflammation, facilitating healing.

Burn and Sunburn Relief – A topical application of St. John's Wort oil can provide soothing relief for burn injuries, including sunburns. The herb's anti-inflammatory compounds help to lessen redness and swelling, while its moisturizing effect prevents peeling and helps to maintain skin hydration.

Eczema and Psoriasis – Additionally, St. John's Wort has been traditionally used to manage symptoms associated with skin conditions like eczema and psoriasis. It can help to soothe itching, reduce inflammation, and promote skin regeneration in affected areas.

Remember that using St. John's Wort oil necessitates a degree of prudence as it can trigger photosensitivity, leading to heightened skin vulnerability to sunlight. It's generally better to apply this oil when the sun has set and to never forget to shield your skin with sunblock during the daytime. Even with natural remedies like this, it's wise to talk with your doctor before starting St. John's Wort, particularly if you're also on other prescribed medications or therapies.

Comfrey

This humble flowering plant, often overlooked, is a powerhouse regarding skin health. Comfrey's most prized component, allantoin, is known for its extraordinary anti-inflammatory and antioxidant prowess and ability to accelerate wound healing. Comfrey can act as your skin's dedicated technician, unflaggingly working to reverse the damage and finetune your skin's texture.

Aloe Vera

Aloe Vera, often called the "plant of immortality" by the Egyptians, is a succulent plant species from the genus Aloe. Its rich history of medicinal use dates back to ancient times, and it has held a prized position in both traditional and modern health practices. Among its myriad applications, aloe vera is especially renowned for its healing effects on skin damage.

Aloe vera leaves contain a clear gel composed of approximately 96% water and a cocktail of beneficial compounds, including vitamins, minerals, amino acids, and antioxidants. But perhaps one of the most remarkable attributes of aloe vera is its ability to soothe and repair damaged skin.

Healing Sunburns – Aloe vera is a common go-to remedy for sunburn. Its potent anti-inflammatory properties help to reduce redness and swelling, while its natural cooling effect provides immediate relief from pain and discomfort. The plant's gel also contains polysaccharides that encourage skin growth and repair, helping to speed up the healing process.

Treating Minor Burns and Cuts – Apart from sunburns, aloe vera has been traditionally used to treat minor burns and cuts. The analgesic properties of aloe help to dull pain, while its antiseptic qualities protect against infection. The aloe vera gel's moisturizing effect also helps prevent skin dryness and accelerates the healing of wounds.

Soothing Skin Irritations – From insect bites and rashes to more chronic conditions like psoriasis and eczema, aloe vera has been used to soothe various skin irritations. Its anti-inflammatory and antimicrobial properties help to reduce itchiness and inflammation, promoting healing and providing relief.

Promoting Healthy Skin Aging – Aloe vera's skin benefits are not confined to damage repair alone. The plant is rich in antioxidants such as vitamins C and E, which fight against skin-damaging free radicals. Regular application of aloe vera gel can help to keep the skin hydrated, reduce the appearance of wrinkles, and maintain the skin's elasticity.

Sea Buckthorn

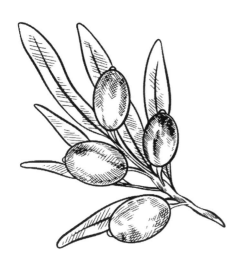

The sea buckthorn, a resilient shrub native to Europe and Asia, has long been valued in traditional medicine. Its Latin name, Hippophae rhamnoides, means "shiny horse," alluding to its historical use for promoting shiny horse coats. Today, every part of this plant, from its bright orange berries to its leaves and bark, is recognized for its impressive health benefits. However, sea buckthorn's potency regarding skin health and healing is most apparent.

Sea buckthorn contains nutrients and bioactive compounds, such as vitamins C and E, carotenoids, flavonoids, and essential fatty acids, including the rare Omega-7. These compounds substantially benefit the skin, making sea buckthorn oil a coveted ingredient in natural skincare.

<u>Healing Skin Damages</u>

Sea buckthorn's potent antioxidant properties make it particularly beneficial for repairing skin damage. Its high vitamin C content supports the synthesis of collagen, a protein that gives the skin its structure and elasticity. This can expedite the healing of wounds, cuts, burns, and other types of skin damage.

The oil derived from sea buckthorn seeds and pulp is rich in Omega-7, a fatty acid for skin health. Studies have found that Omega-7 can enhance skin regeneration and reduce inflammation, thus promoting the healing process and reducing the likelihood of scar formation.

Furthermore, the carotenoids in sea buckthorn can protect the skin against UV radiation, one of the leading causes of skin damage. By absorbing and scattering harmful UV rays, these compounds can prevent sunburn and mitigate the long-term damage associated with excessive sun exposure.

Sea buckthorn oil can be applied topically to the skin to assist in healing. Due to its intense pigmentation, it should be used sparingly, and it's always advisable to perform a patch test first to ensure there's no allergic reaction. Sea buckthorn oil can be found in many skincare products or used in its pure form, often diluted with a carrier oil.

Herbal Skincare Routine

Remember those mornings when the mirror reflects a shiny forehead or those winter days when no amount of moisturizer seems to quench your skin's thirst? We all have different skin types, and each type calls for a unique care routine. This chapter helps you understand whether your skin leans more toward being oily, dry, combination, or sensitive and how to nourish it with herbal goodness. We'll be exploring the lush gardens of nature's pharmacy, choosing the right herbs that work wonders on your specific skin type.

With decades of experience in the herbal realm, I recall the first time that I made a face wash from chamomile and honey - a life-changing moment that sparked a deep love for herbal remedies. It was a delight for my sensitive skin and a divine revelation of what nature can offer us. Inspired by this, we will be whipping up some DIY herbal skincare recipes - everything from face washes, toners, and moisturizers, to face masks.

Your Daily Routine

To achieve healthier, happier skin, all it takes is a simple three-step skincare routine: cleanse, tone, and moisturize. With a touch of herbal magic, you can enhance the effectiveness of these steps and nourish your skin from within.

Herbal Cleansing

Cleansing your skin is akin to setting a clean canvas, preparing your skin for the following nurturing. Commercial face washes can be harsh, stripping away your skin's natural oils. Why not replace them with something gentle yet effective, like a herbal cleanser?

Enter your first companion on this journey: chamomile. It's a gentle herb that soothes and cleanses your skin. Blend chamomile tea with honey for a mild cleanser that refreshes your skin. Also, try lavender or rosemary, known for their cleaning properties.

Toning with Herbs

Toning is an often-ignored step in skincare. A good toner balances your skin's pH and prepares it for moisturization. Toners have the function of bridging the gap between cleansing and moisturizing.

To create your herbal toner, witch hazel makes a fantastic choice, especially for oily and acne-prone skin. A green tea toner could work wonders for those with normal or combination skin. If your skin tends toward dryness, a rosewater toner could be your best bet.

Herbal Moisturizing

Now it's time to lock in the goodness with a moisturizer. A great moisturizer does more than just seal the deal - it nourishes your skin and leaves it soft and supple.

You can moisturize your skin with aloe vera and a few drops of lavender essential oil. It's a soothing, nourishing treat for all skin types. A dab of coconut oil with a touch of chamomile can work like magic, especially for dry skin.

This simple three-step routine is a starting point. But remember, the charm of an herbal skincare routine is its flexibility. Feel free to mix and match the herbs as you get more comfortable with their properties.

Different Skin Types

Just as people have different personalities, our skin has unique quirks and characteristics. To fully embrace the benefits of herbal skincare, it's important to understand your skin type and its different needs with the changing seasons. Let's delve into this exciting exploration.

Oily Skin

Picture yourself standing by a glistening stream on a warm sunny day - that's what oily skin often feels like. It's shiny, slightly greasy to the touch, and often accompanied by enlarged pores. But on the bright side, oily skin is generally more resilient and less prone to wrinkling.

For those with an oilier skin type, astringent herbs like witch hazel, sage, and lemongrass are true allies. They help control oil production without over-drying your skin. A tea tree oil diluted in a carrier oil like jojoba is great for oily skin, given its antibacterial and anti-inflammatory properties.

Dry Skin

Imagine a beautiful, arid desert that's dry skin. It's prone to tightness, rough patches, and visible lines. This skin type yearns for deep hydration and nourishment.

Herbs like calendula, chamomile, and lavender are wonderfully beneficial for dry skin due to their moisturizing and soothing properties. Add some of these to a hydrating base like shea butter or almond oil, and you'll get a lush, natural moisturizer.

Combination Skin

And the enigma of combination skin - oily in some places (usually the T-zone), dry in others. The trick here is balance. You need to hydrate the dry parts without overwhelming the oily ones.

A mix of herbs can help here. Green tea, known for its balancing properties, could be an excellent addition to your skincare routine. You could also use witch hazel on the oilier parts and calendula on the drier ones.

Sensitive Skin

Sensitive skin is like a delicate wildflower. It may react to new products or ingredients, turning red, itchy, or inflamed. Gentle care is the key here.

Choose mild, soothing herbs such as chamomile, calendula, and aloe vera for sensitive skin. They're gentle and often help calm inflammation and redness.

Seasonal Skincare

Beyond individual skin types, our skin's needs can change with the seasons. Let's see how we can adapt our herbal skincare routine to these seasonal shifts.

In the **summer**, our skin tends to be oilier. So you must go for lighter, astringent herbs such as witch hazel or green tea. As for the **winter**, our skin often leans toward dryness. This is the time to whip out those hydrating herbs like calendula and oils like shea butter or almond oil.

During **spring**, when everything is in bloom, some may experience heightened skin sensitivity due to allergies. Sticking to more gentle herbs like chamomile during this time is best. And in **autumn**, as the air gets drier, consider incorporating more hydrating elements into your skincare routine to help your skin adjust.

The versatility of herbal skincare is what makes it amazing. With an assortment of herbs at your disposal, you can customize your skincare regimen to suit your skin's specific needs. Let's keep in mind that everyone's skin is unique, and what works for one person might not for another. So, listen to your skin, take note of its response to different herbs, and feel free to experiment.

Chapter Three
DIY Recipes

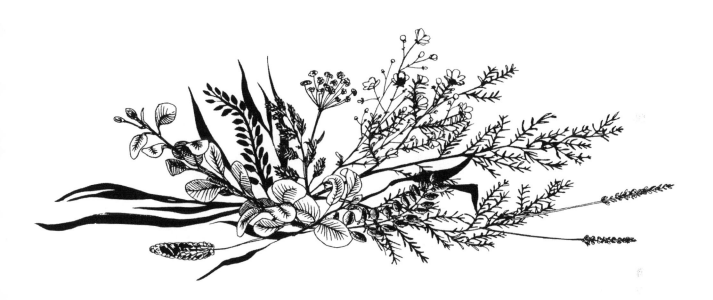

The joy of crafting your skincare products is a sensory experience, with your hands touching the fresh, earthy herbs, your nose taking in their intoxicating aromas, and your skin eagerly awaiting the love it's about to receive. There's something wonderfully satisfying about seeing your handmade creations lined up on your bathroom shelf, knowing and smelling every ingredient that went into them.

So, ready to get your hands dirty and your skin a lot cleaner? Let's explore these DIY herbal skincare recipes.

Face Wash

Chamomile and Honey Face Wash

Properties: Chamomile is known for its calming and anti-inflammatory properties, while honey is a natural antibacterial and humectant, which helps to cleanse and moisturize the skin.

Ingredients:

- 1 cup chamomile tea (cooled)

- 1 tablespoon raw honey

- 1 tablespoon liquid castile soap

Instructions:

1. Brew a cup of chamomile tea and allow it to cool.

2. Mix the cooled tea, raw honey, and liquid castile soap in a bowl.

3. Pour the mixture into a clean bottle.

Prep Time: 10-15 minutes

If stored properly, you can keep the Chamomile and Honey Face Wash for about 1 to 2 weeks. It is recommended to store it in a cool, dry place and use a clean bottle with a tight lid to prevent contamination. However, since this is a homemade product without preservatives, its shelf life may vary depending on temperature and storage conditions. It's always a good idea to observe any changes in texture, color, or odor, and if you notice any signs of spoilage, it's best to discard the face wash and make a fresh batch.

Tip: Shake the bottle before each use, as the ingredients may separate over time.

Green Tea and Aloe Vera Face Wash

Properties: Green tea is rich in antioxidants, reducing inflammation and oiliness. Aloe Vera is soothing and hydrating.

Ingredients:

- 1/2 cup brewed green tea (cooled)

- 1/2 cup aloe vera gel

- 1 tablespoon liquid castile soap

Instructions:

1. Mix the cooled green tea, aloe vera gel, and liquid castile soap in a bowl.

2. Pour the mixture into a clean pump bottle.

Prep Time: 10-15 minutes

Tip: Use within a week or store in the refrigerator for a cooling cleanse.

Lavender and Oatmeal Face Wash

Properties: Lavender is calming and anti-inflammatory, while oatmeal soothes and gently exfoliates.

Ingredients:

- 1/4 cup ground oats

- 1/8 cup liquid castile soap

- 1/8 cup water

- 5-7 drops of lavender essential oil

Instructions:

1. Mix ground oats, liquid castile soap, water, and lavender essential oil in a bowl.

2. Store the mixture in a jar.

Prep Time: 5 minutes

This facewash can be safely stored for approximately 1 to 2 weeks. Please keep it in a cool, dry place and a tightly sealed jar. As a homemade product without preservatives, its shelf life may vary depending on storage conditions. However, it's best to monitor any changes in texture, color, or odor and discard the face wash if signs of spoilage are observed.

Tip: Wet your face before applying this face wash. It's a gentle exfoliator, so scrub lightly!

Rosewater and Glycerin Face Wash

Properties: Rosewater is refreshing and balancing, while glycerin is a humectant that attracts moisture to the skin.

Ingredients:

- 1/2 cup rosewater

- 1/4 cup liquid castile soap

- 1 tablespoon vegetable glycerin

Instructions:

1. Combine rosewater, liquid castile soap, and vegetable glycerin in a bowl.

2. Pour the mixture into a clean bottle.

Prep Time: 5 minutes

This product can typically be stored for about 1 to 2 weeks. It is recommended to keep it in a cool, dry place and use a clean bottle with a tight lid to maintain its freshness.

Tip: This face wash is perfect for combination skin as rosewater helps balance oil production.

Witch Hazel and Tea Tree Face Wash

Properties: Witch hazel acts as an astringent, helping to tighten the skin and reduce inflammation. Tea tree oil is antibacterial and great for combatting acne.

Ingredients:

- 1/2 cup witch hazel

- 1/4 cup liquid castile soap

- 10 drops of tea tree essential oil

Instructions:

1. Mix the witch hazel, liquid castile soap, and tea tree essential oil in a bowl.

2. Pour the mixture into a clean bottle.

Prep Time: 5 minutes

When stored appropriately in a cool, dry place with a tightly sealed bottle, this facewash can typically be stored for 1 to 2 weeks.

Tip: If your skin feels dry after using this face wash, reduce the amount of witch hazel. It's beneficial for oily skin types.

Toner

Rosewater and Green Tea Toner

Properties: Rosewater helps maintain the skin's pH balance, has anti-inflammatory properties, and aids in removing oil and dirt. Green tea is rich in antioxidants, reducing inflammation and oiliness.

Ingredients:

- 1 cup green tea (cooled)

- 1/2 cup rosewater

Instructions:

1. Brew a cup of green tea and let it cool.

2. Mix the cooled green tea with rosewater in a clean spray bottle.

Prep Time: 15 minutes (including cooling time)

Properly stored in a cool, dry place and in a clean spray bottle, this toner can typically be preserved for approximately 1 to 2 weeks.

Tips: Spray this toner directly onto your face for a refreshing and hydrating boost throughout the day.

Witch Hazel and Lavender Toner

Witch hazel helps minimize pores and inflammation, and lavender has calming and anti-inflammatory properties.

Ingredients:

- 1/2 cup witch hazel

- 1/2 cup distilled water

- 10 drops of lavender essential oil

Instructions:

1. Mix witch hazel, distilled water, and lavender essential oil in a clean bottle.

2. Shake well to combine.

Prep Time: 5 minutes

When stored properly in a cool, dry place, this toner can be kept for approximately 1 to 2 weeks. It is recommended to use a clean bottle for storage and make sure the lid is tightly sealed.

Tip: Apply using a cotton pad after cleansing. Keep away from the eye area.

Apple Cider Vinegar and Chamomile Toner

Properties: Apple cider vinegar helps balance your skin's pH levels and remove excess oils. Chamomile is soothing and anti-inflammatory.

Ingredients:

- 1/2 cup chamomile tea (cooled)

- 1/2 cup apple cider vinegar

Instructions:

1. Brew a cup of chamomile tea and allow it to cool.

2. Combine the cooled chamomile tea and apple cider vinegar in a clean bottle.

Prep Time: 15 minutes (including cooling time)

If stored properly in a cool, dry place using a tightly sealed, clean bottle, the toner should stay good for around 1 to 2 weeks. Just keep an eye out for any changes in smell, color, or texture, and if it starts to go bad, it's best to toss it out.

Tip: If you have sensitive skin, dilute the apple cider vinegar with more chamomile tea.

Aloe Vera and Cucumber Toner

Properties: Aloe Vera is moisturizing and soothing, while cucumber is hydrating and helps to reduce puffiness.

Ingredients:

- 1/2 cup aloe vera juice

- 1/2 cup cucumber juice

Instructions:

1. Extract the juice from a cucumber.

2. Mix the cucumber juice and aloe vera juice in a clean spray bottle.

Prep Time: 10 minutes

If you store it right, you can keep this toner for 1 to 2 weeks. Just make sure to keep it in a cool, dry place and use a clean spray bottle.

Tip: Store this toner in the refrigerator for a refreshing, cooling effect. Great for use after a day in the sun!

Moisturizer

Shea Butter and Chamomile Moisturizer

Properties: Shea butter is deeply moisturizing and rich in vitamins A and E. Chamomile is soothing and anti-inflammatory.

Ingredients:

- 1/2 cup shea butter

- 1/4 cup jojoba oil

- 1/4 cup dried chamomile flowers

Instructions:

1. Melt the shea butter in a double boiler.

2. Add jojoba oil and chamomile flowers to the melted shea butter and let it infuse on low heat for 1 hour.

3. Strain the mixture and let it cool.

4. Once cooled, whip the mixture until it achieves a creamy consistency.

5. Store in a clean jar.

Prep Time: 1 hour 15 minutes

Tip: This moisturizer is perfect for dry skin. Apply it while your skin is still damp for maximum absorption.

Coconut Oil and Green Tea Moisturizer

Properties: Coconut oil is deeply moisturizing and has antibacterial properties. Green tea is rich in antioxidants and helps reduce inflammation.

Ingredients:

- 1/2 cup coconut oil

- 2 tablespoons loose green tea

Instructions:

1. Melt the coconut oil in a double boiler, then add the green tea.

2. Let the green tea infuse on low heat for 1 hour.

3. Strain the oil, squeezing out all the goodness from the tea leaves.

4. Let the oil solidify, then whip it up into a creamy consistency.

5. Store in a clean jar.

Prep Time: 1 hour 15 minutes

Tips: This moisturizer has a longer shelf life due to coconut oil's antimicrobial properties. It's great for those with oily skin or acne-prone skin.

Cocoa Butter and Lavender Moisturizer

Cocoa butter is a luxurious moisturizer packed with nourishing fatty acids that deeply hydrate and replenish the skin. Lavender, on the other hand, has a soothing effect and helps to reduce inflammation, adding to the overall calming benefits of this skincare ingredient combination.

Ingredients:

- 1/2 cup cocoa butter

- 1/4 cup sweet almond oil

- 10 drops of lavender essential oil

Instructions:

1. Melt the cocoa butter in a double boiler.

2. Once melted, remove from heat and mix in sweet almond oil and lavender essential oil.

3. Allow the mixture to cool and solidify slightly, then whip until creamy.

4. Store in a clean jar.

Prep Time: 20 minutes

Tips: This rich moisturizer is perfect for dry skin or winter use.

Aloe Vera and Almond Oil Moisturizer

Properties: Aloe Vera provides moisturization and soothing properties, while almond oil deeply hydrates and is abundant in vitamin E, ensuring your skin stays soft and supple.

Ingredients:

- 1/2 cup pure aloe vera gel

- 1/4 cup almond oil

- 10 drops of lavender essential oil

Instructions:

1. Whisk together aloe vera gel, almond oil, and lavender essential oil in a bowl.

2. Store the mixture in a clean jar.

Prep Time: 5 minutes

Tip: This is a lightweight moisturizer, perfect for oily skin or for use during the summer.

Olive Oil and Rosemary Moisturizer

Olive oil is rich in antioxidants and hydrating squalene, making it superb for the skin. Rosemary has natural antiseptic properties, which help remove impurities from the skin.

Ingredients:

- 1/2 cup olive oil

- 1/4 cup beeswax pellets

- 1/4 cup rosemary-infused water (cooled)

Instructions:

1. Melt the beeswax in a double boiler

2. Once melted, remove from heat and slowly add olive oil, stirring constantly.

3. Gradually add the rosemary-infused water, and keep stirring until the mixture cools and thickens.

4. Pour the mixture into a clean jar before it fully solidifies.

5. Allow the mixture to cool completely and set.

Prep Time: 30 minutes

Tips: This moisturizer is a perfect all-rounder, suitable for all skin types. Remember to patch test if you have sensitive skin, for some people can react to rosemary.

Face Mask

Turmeric and Honey Face Mask

Properties: Turmeric has anti-inflammatory and antioxidant properties, and honey is moisturizing and antibacterial.

Ingredients:

- 1 teaspoon turmeric powder

- 1 tablespoon raw honey

Instructions:

    1. Mix turmeric powder and raw honey in a bowl.

    2. Apply the mixture to your clean face and leave it on for 15-20 minutes.

    3. Rinse off with warm water.

Prep Time: 5 minutes

Tips: Turmeric can stain your skin temporarily. To avoid this, you can use a gentle facial cleanser after rinsing off the mask.

Aloe Vera and Green Tea Face Mask

Aloe Vera is soothing and hydrating, while green tea is antioxidant-rich and helps reduce inflammation.

Ingredients:

- 2 tablespoons aloe vera gel

- 1 tablespoon green tea leaves (or green tea bag content)

Instructions:

    1. Mix aloe vera gel and green tea leaves in a bowl.

    2. Apply the mixture to your face and leave it on for 15-20 minutes.

    3. Rinse off with cool water.

Prep Time: 5 minutes

Tip: This mask is particularly soothing after a day in the sun.

Oatmeal and Chamomile Face Mask

Oatmeal is soothing and offers gentle exfoliation, while chamomile is known for its calming properties and anti-inflammatory benefits.

Ingredients:

- 1/2 cup ground oats

- 1/2 cup chamomile tea (cooled)

Instructions:

    1. Mix ground oats with chamomile tea to create a paste.

2. Apply the paste to your face and let it sit for 10-15 minutes.

3. Rinse with warm water.

Prep Time: 10 minutes (including cooling time)

Tip: You can add a bit of honey for extra moisturization.

Rosewater and Clay Face Mask

Properties: Rosewater helps maintain the skin's pH balance, has anti-inflammatory properties, and aids in removing oil and dirt. Clay is excellent for drawing out impurities and excess oil.

Ingredients:

- 2 tablespoons clay (e.g., kaolin for sensitive skin, bentonite for oilier skin)

- Enough rosewater to form a paste

Instructions:

1. Mix the clay and rosewater in a bowl to form a smooth paste.

2. Apply the mask to your face and let it dry (about 10-15 minutes).

3. Rinse off with warm water.

Prep Time: 5 minutes

Tips: Apply a moisturizer after this mask, as clay can dry out your skin. Avoid using metal utensils with bentonite clay as it can react and reduce its effectiveness.

Patch Testing & Safety Precautions

When it comes to using herbal skincare products, it's essential to take some safety precautions. Just like embarking on any new adventure, it's wise to approach it cautiously.

One crucial step is performing a patch test. It's like introducing your skin to a new friend. Find a small, inconspicuous area on your skin, such as your forearm or behind your ear. Apply a tiny amount of the product and wait for 24 hours. If there's no reaction, you're good to go! But if you experience itching, redness, swelling, or discomfort, wash it off immediately and avoid using that ingredient on your face or larger skin areas.

Remember, even seemingly harmless herbs can cause allergies in some people. So, it's better to be safe than sorry. Patch testing helps avoid potential skin reactions and ensures a smooth skincare journey.

Here are some safety guidelines because, remember, even superheroes have their weaknesses:

1. **Pregnancy:** Some herbs, like sage and rosemary, can stimulate uterine contractions, so they're best avoided during pregnancy. Always consult with a healthcare provider or herbalist if you're pregnant or breastfeeding.

2. **Photosensitivity:** Certain herbs, like St. John's Wort and some citrus essential oils, can make your skin more sensitive to sunlight, leading to quicker burns or rashes. If a product makes your skin photosensitive, wear adequate sun protection or use it in your nighttime routine.

3. **Pre-existing conditions:** If you have a skin-related health condition, some herbs might interfere with your treatments or exacerbate symptoms. For instance, those with eczema or rosacea might find essential oils irritating. A healthcare provider can guide you on the safe use of herbs in such cases.

4. **Medication Interactions:** If you're on medication, some herbs could potentially interact with them. For instance, Ginkgo Biloba is a popular herb that can interfere with anticoagulants, leading to a higher risk of bleeding. Always check with your healthcare provider if you're on any medication.

5. **Quality:** Ensure your herbs are good quality, organic, and free from pesticides or other contaminants.

The world of herbal skincare is vast and varied, and there's something suitable for everyone. While it may seem there's a lot to watch out for, don't be deterred. Always listen to your skin—it's the best guide to herbal mastery.

Consider the tale of my friend, Sarah. She excitedly jumped into the realm of herbal skincare without patch testing first. As fate would have it, she had a mild allergic reaction to chamomile, usually a very soothing herb. It wasn't severe, but it was a wake-up call about the importance of patch testing and safety. Since then, she's learned her lesson and enjoyed many other herbs that agree with her skin.

So, dear readers, venture forth with this wisdom in your pocket. Listen to your skin, observe, learn, and enjoy this beautiful adventure. Safety comes first, but fun follows closely behind in the vibrant world of herbal skincare.

BOOK VI

GROWING AND FORAGING YOUR OWN HERBS

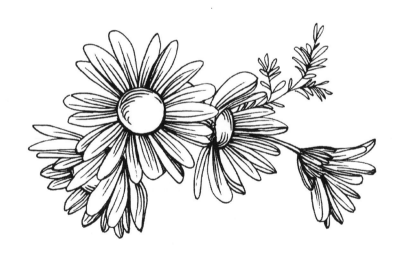

AMBER WHITMORE

Introduction

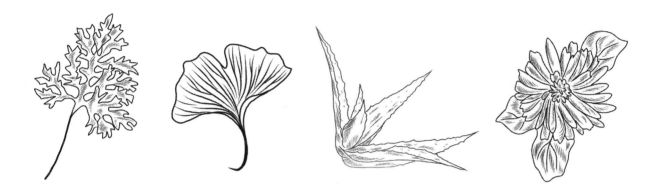

Planting a seed, watching it develop, and then using what you've grown to better your health and well-being is immensely empowering.

This book will teach you how to become a green-thumbed herbalist capable of cultivating your therapeutic sanctuary right in your garden. We'll look at the art and science of planning and building a medicinal herb garden, where functionality and beauty coexist, and every plant has a purpose.

Then, we'll go through climatic concerns, matching the proper herbs to your individual weather circumstances and assuring a prosperous and healthy herbal bounty. From there, you'll be armed with advice on planting, caring for, and maintaining your herbs, ensuring they thrive from seedling to full bloom.

And finally, as the fruits of your labor unfold, we'll guide you through harvesting and preserving your herbs, sealing in their potent benefits throughout the year. So, let's roll up our sleeves and let our hands touch the earth as we explore the captivating world of herb gardening.

Chapter One
Green Thumb Healing

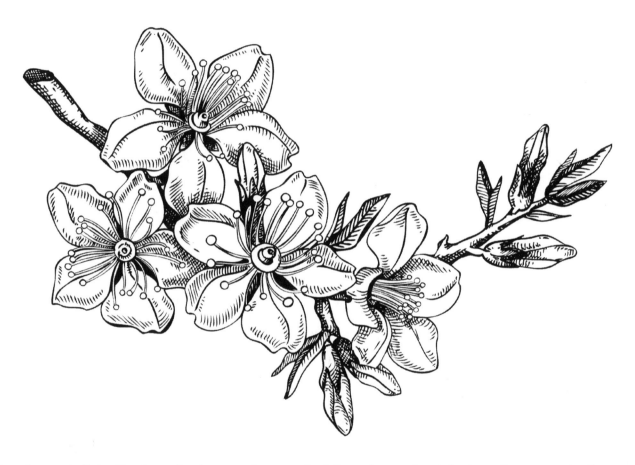

Creating a medicinal herb garden is not only a worthwhile endeavor, but it is also a fun one, as it allows you to cultivate and nurture your health right in your own backyard. This project combines the aesthetic benefits of gardening with the health-promoting properties of medicinal herbs, making it a rewarding experience. A successful medicinal herb garden, like any other enterprise, requires careful planning and design.

Planning Your Medicinal Herb Garden: A 7-Step Guide

Step 1: Define Your Intent

Before starting, it's crucial to identify the primary purpose of your medicinal herb garden. Are you looking to grow herbs for teas or culinary uses, or are you more focused on their medicinal properties for specific health concerns? Are you drawn to the healing power of plants, or do you simply want to beautify your outdoor space while also growing useful herbs? Understanding your garden's purpose will serve as the guiding compass, informing the types of herbs you choose and the design of your garden.

Step 2: Pinpoint the Perfect Location

The next step is to select an appropriate location for your garden. Most medicinal herbs thrive in full sun, meaning at least six hours of sunlight each day, while others tolerate partial shade. Examine your available space; remember it doesn't have to be large. A sunny balcony, a small backyard, or even a window sill can serve as a mini medicinal herb garden. Also, consider the soil quality - a well-draining soil enriched with organic matter is ideal for most herbs.

Step 3: Draft a Garden Blueprint

After choosing a location, put your design ideas onto paper. This doesn't require professional architectural skills but a simple sketch or outline of your garden layout. Consider the space needed for each plant to grow and spread. Some herbs, like mint, can be vigorous and may need containment to prevent them from taking over the garden. Design pathways to ensure you have easy access to all plants when it's time for harvesting.

Step 4: Select Suitable Herbs

The fourth step is the most exciting one - selecting your herbs! When making your choices, take into account your original purpose, the climate of your area, and the specific growing requirements of each herb. Starting with a mix of easy-to-grow annuals and perennials is a good approach. Consider familiar herbs like chamomile, mint, sage, and rosemary, but don't shy away from incorporating more exotic herbs that pique your interest.

Step 5: Prepare the Garden Bed

With the design ready and herbs selected, it's time to roll up your sleeves and prepare your garden bed. Clear the chosen area of weeds and other debris. If you're planting directly in the ground, improve the soil condition by adding organic compost, providing the plants with essential nutrients. If you're using pots or planters, ensure they have adequate drainage holes and are filled with a quality potting mix.

Step 6: Planting Your Chosen Herbs

Finally, the time has come to bring life to your garden by planting your chosen herbs. You can start herbs from seeds, propagate them from cuttings, or buy small plants from a nursery. Each herb comes with its own set of planting guidelines, including the recommended planting depth, spacing, and watering requirements. By following these instructions, you can ensure that your herbs thrive and grow robustly.

Step 7: Nurturing and Watching Your Garden Grow

Creating a medicinal herb garden is an ongoing journey, not a one-time task. Patience, nurturing, and a keen eye are needed to care for your herbs, spot potential issues, and manage them quickly. Over time, your role transitions from being a gardener to a custodian, watching over your garden and helping it flourish. The end result—a thriving garden filled with healing plants—is truly rewarding and worth the effort.

Selecting the Right Herbs for Your Climate

Choosing the right herbs for your garden is a delightful task, but it's not solely based on personal preference. You need to consider your local climate and the specific growing needs of each herb. If you reside in a region with long, harsh winters, tender tropical herbs like lemongrass might struggle, while hardy herbs like thyme or sage could thrive.

Imagine me in my early gardening days, eager to grow all sorts of exotic herbs I had read about. I soon realized that some plants couldn't handle my local climate. Trial and error taught me a valuable lesson: the importance of climate considerations when choosing herbs.

Start by understanding your **USDA hardiness zone**, which provides a guide to the types of plants that can grow in your area based on the average minimum winter temperature.

The USDA Hardiness Zone Map is a tool developed by the United States Department of Agriculture (USDA) to help gardeners and growers identify which plants most likely thrive in their specific geographic location. The map is based on the average annual minimum winter temperature, divided into 10-degree Fahrenheit zones.

The map is color-coded and divided into 13 primary zones, each representing a range of winter temperatures. Each zone is further divided into "a" and "b" to provide a more precise understanding of the climate, making a total of 26 unique zones across the map.

For instance, if you live in Zone 6, the average annual minimum winter temperature is -10 to 0 degrees Fahrenheit. If you're in Zone 6a, the temperature range would be -10 to -5 degrees Fahrenheit, while in Zone 6b, it would be -5 to 0 degrees Fahrenheit.

Now, let's explore some herbs and their ideal climates.

Tropical Herbs

Tropical herbs can be quite thirsty, so keep their soil consistently moist but not waterlogged. You might find it helpful to add some compost or well-rotted manure to your soil to improve its water-holding capacity and provide nutrients for your plants.

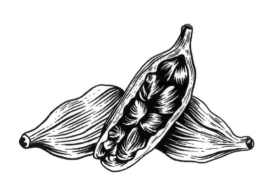

Cardamom

Cardamom (Elettaria cardamomum): Cardamom is a tropical plant that thrives in humid and warm conditions. The plant may grow up to 10 feet tall and has gorgeous, big leaves, making it an aesthetically pleasing plant. It is an aromatic spice used in savory and sweet recipes, particularly in Indian and Middle Eastern cuisine.

Lemongrass (Cymbopogon citratus): This tropical herb thrives in hot and humid climates, soaking up full sun and well-drained soil. It's a tall, perennial grass with a fresh, lemony aroma and is commonly used in Asian cuisine, particularly Thai and Viet-namese dishes. Lemongrass can grow up to 5 feet tall, requiring some space. If you're in a cooler climate, consider growing lemongrass in a large pot that can be moved indoors during winter. It's a resilient herb and can usually bounce back if affected by a cold snap. A fun fact about lemongrass is that it's a natural mosquito repellent, making it a great addition to a patio or outdoor seating area.

Ginger (Zingiber officinale): Ginger enjoys the warm, humid climate of the tropics. It grows from rhizomes (underground stems), which can be bought at a garden shop or supermarket. Choose a piece with many eye buds (similar to potato eyes), as these may grow new plants. Ginger likes filtered sunlight, so a location beneath a tree or on a porch with bright, indirect lighting is wonderful. If you live in a colder climate, you can plant ginger in a container and bring it indoors for the winter. Ginger takes about 8-10 months to grow, but the wait is well worth it when you can harvest fresh ginger.

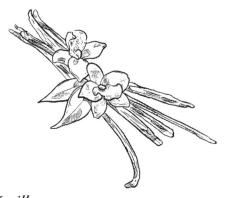

Vanilla

Turmeric (Curcuma longa): Like ginger, turmeric is a tropical plant that grows from rhizomes. It prefers warm, humid conditions and rich, well-drained soil. Turmeric plants have large, decorative leaves and can grow up to 3 feet tall, making them an attractive addition to your garden or indoor plant collection. If you're in a colder climate, turmeric can be grown in a pot and brought indoors over winter. Remember, turmeric takes about 8-10 months to mature!

Vanilla (Vanilla planifolia): Vanilla is a vining orchid native to tropical climates. It's most famous for producing vanilla beans used to make vanilla extract. The plant prefers high humidity and indirect light, making it an excellent choice for an indoor plant if you can provide these conditions. Growing vanilla and getting it to produce beans can be a bit complex and time-consuming, but it's an exciting challenge for the more adventurous gardener.

A handy tip for growing these herbs indoors during winter is to place them near a window where they will receive plenty of indirect sunlight, and consider using a humidity tray or a room humidifier to mimic the humid conditions they love.

Mint, Lemon Balm, and Chives

Remember that all these herbs appreciate well-drained soil and regular watering. However, be careful not to overwater, as this can lead to root rot. A good rule of thumb is to water when the top inch of soil feels dry to the touch.

Mint (Mentha): Mint is a robust herb that can quickly adapt to various climates, from temperate to tropical. It prefers a spot with partial shade, although it can also handle full sun if given enough moisture. Mint is known for its rapid growth; it can quickly spread through your garden, so many gardeners plant it in a container to keep it under control. You can enjoy its refreshing flavor in teas, salads, or as a garnish in various dishes. A bonus is its wonderful aroma that can fill your garden every time you brush past it.

Chives (Allium schoenoprasum): Chives are perennial plants that do well in various climates. They prefer full sun but can tolerate partial shade. They're easy to grow, requiring only well-drained soil and regular watering. With their mild onion-like flavor, chives are a great addition to salads, egg dishes, and soups. Their purple flowers are attractive and can bring a splash of color to your garden.

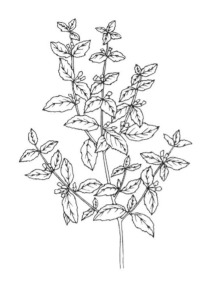

Lemon Balm | Melissa

Lemon Balm (Melissa officinalis): Lemon balm is a hardy perennial herb that can tolerate various climates. It prefers well-drained soil, and while it can grow in full sun, it does appreciate a bit of afternoon shade in hotter climates. Lemon balm is beloved for its lemon-scented leaves that can be used in teas, salads, or flavor dishes. It's also known for its calming properties and can be used in herbal remedies to promote relaxation and reduce stress.

A fun fact about mint and lemon balm is that they are known to repel certain pests, so planting them around your garden can serve a dual purpose - providing you with delicious herbs and protecting your other plants.

As for the vigorous growth of mint, consider using it as a ground cover in areas where you'd like to suppress weeds. Just be ready to cut it back if it starts invading areas it's not wanted. Alternatively, as mentioned earlier, growing mint in a container is a great way to enjoy this refreshing herb without worrying about it taking over your garden.

Mediterranean Herbs

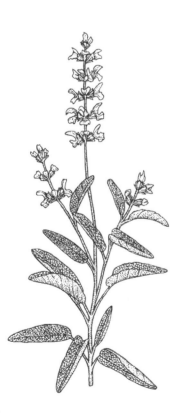

Sage

Mediterranean herbs, like Sage, Rosemary, Lavender, and Thyme, are sun-loving plants that thrive best in hot, dry conditions reminiscent of their native habitats. These herbs are beloved not just for their culinary uses but also for their aromatic qualities and resilience in challenging weather conditions.

Sage (Salvia officinalis): Sage is a hardy perennial that enjoys plenty of sunshine and light, well-drained soil. It has aromatic, grayish-green leaves that add a potent flavor to many dishes. For beginners, it's a low-maintenance herb that requires little attention once established. Sage can be easily propagated from cuttings, so you can share your sage plant with friends or even expand your garden.

Rosemary (Rosmarinus officinalis): Rosemary is a fragrant evergreen herb well-suited to hot, dry climates. It prefers well-drained soil and can handle a bit of neglect when it comes to watering. In fact, overwatering is one of the most common ways to accidentally harm your rosemary plant. When planting rosemary, give it plenty of space, as it can grow quite large.

Lavender (Lavandula): The key to a happy lavender plant is good drainage and lots of sunshine. Lavender is drought-resistant once established and prefers infrequent, deep watering to frequent, shallow watering. Bees love lavender flowers, and they make an excellent addition to homemade cosmetics or as a calming tea ingredient.

Thyme (Thymus vulgaris): Thyme is a small, creeping plant that thrives in full sun and well-drained soil. It's a fantastic herb for rock gardens or as a ground cover in sunny spots. Thyme comes in many varieties, each with a unique flavor and aroma, from lemon to the traditional English thyme.

Tip #1 - Mediterranean herbs often have fine, sandy soil in their native habitat, which allows water to drain quickly. If your garden soil is heavy clay or tends to stay soggy, consider adding sand or fine gravel to improve drainage or plant your herbs in raised beds or pots. Remember, these herbs are adapted to a dry climate and can often do well with less water than you might think. Overwatering can lead to root rot and other diseases.

Tip #2 - these herbs are not just practical, but they're also beautiful. Sage's grey-green leaves, rosemary's tall, sturdy posture, lavender's fragrant purple blooms, and thyme's carpet of tiny leaves and flowers can turn your herb garden into a feast for the eyes!

Cold-Hardy Herbs

These herbs are fantastic options for gardeners living in cooler climates. Not only can they tolerate frost and cold temperatures, but they're also low-maintenance, robust, and bring a splash of color to your garden even when the mercury dips.

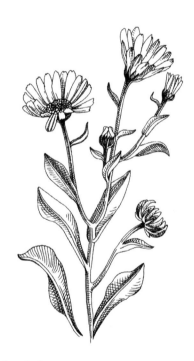

Calendula

Calendula (Calendula officinalis): With its vibrant orange or yellow flowers, calendula is a resilient herb that can handle cooler weather conditions. Its flowers are beautiful, edible, and have various medicinal uses. As a bonus, calendula self-seeds readily, meaning you'll enjoy a recurring bloom of vibrant flowers year after year. Calendula can be used in a range of applications, from salads and soups to skin care products, thanks to its skin-soothing properties.

Echinacea (Echinacea purpurea): Echinacea, commonly known as the purple coneflower, is a perennial plant that's resistant to most pests and diseases. Its vibrant, purple-pink flowers bloom mid to late summer, attracting butterflies and bees to your garden. Echinacea is also renowned for its immune-boosting properties and is a staple in many herbal remedies. As a beginner, you'll appreciate that echinacea is easy to grow from seed or transplants and, once established, can endure drought-like conditions, making it a fuss-free option for your garden.

Horseradish (Armoracia rusticana): This is a robust, cold-tolerant perennial herb grown for its pungent root. The roots are usually harvested in the fall or early spring and are known for their spicy flavor and potential health benefits, including antibacterial properties. While it can become invasive if not managed, horseradish can be an excellent addition to your garden.*Chamomile (Matricaria chamomilla)*: Known for its delicate, daisy-like flowers and calming properties, chamomile is a cold-hardy herb that can withstand cooler temperatures. It prefers full sun but can tolerate partial shade, and it's relatively easy to grow, making it a great choice for beginners. Chamomile flowers can be harvested and dried in teas, tinctures, and skincare products.

To get the most out of these cold-hardy herbs, ensure they have well-drained soil and full sun to partial shade. A fun fact: All these herbs are drought-tolerant once established. This means they're great choices if you're looking to create a low-water garden or 'xeriscape.'

Chapter Two
From Soil to Harvest

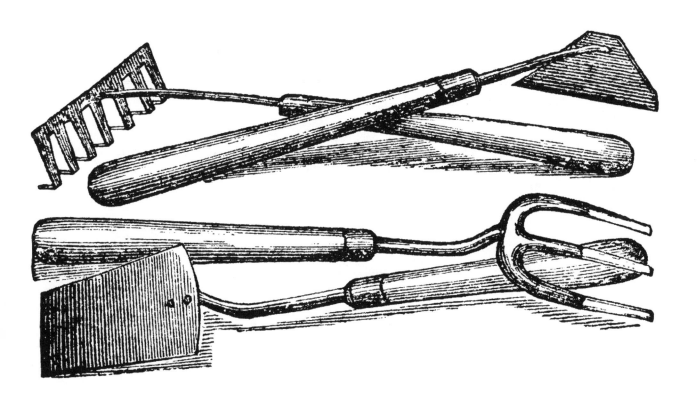

Planting your medicinal herb garden is where the real fun begins! After all the research, planning, and preparation, it's finally time to get your hands dirty.

Every herb has its specific needs regarding soil type, sunlight, and watering. Some herbs like it dry and sunny, while others prefer a bit of shade and moisture. It's essential to group plants with similar needs together. For example, Mediterranean herbs like rosemary and lavender love the sun and well-drained soil. In contrast, herbs like mint and lemon balm prefer more moisture and can handle some shade.

Planting, Care, and Maintenance Tips

Preparing the Soil

Your soil is the foundation of your garden. It provides your plants with the nutrients they need to grow and thrive. For most herbs, well-draining soil is crucial. Adding organic matter like compost or well-rotted manure can improve soil drainage. A general-purpose potting mix should do the trick if you're planting in pots.

Planting Your Herbs

When it comes to planting, there are two routes you can take: seeds or seedlings. Starting from seed is a more cost-effective approach, and it gives you a wider variety of herbs to choose from. However, it also requires more time and patience.

If you choose seeds, follow the planting instructions on the seed packet. Generally, seeds should be planted at a depth approximately three times their size. Cover the seeds with soil, water them gently, and keep the soil moist until the seedlings emerge.

On the other hand, starting with seedlings or small plants can give you a head start. Dig a hole wide and deep enough to accommodate the root ball when planting seedlings. Place the plant in the hole, ensuring the top of the root ball is level with the soil surface. Backfill the hole with soil, gently firm it around the plant's base, and water thoroughly.

Spacing Your Herbs

When growing your herbs, proper spacing is fundamental. Overcrowding can result in inadequate air circulation, which raises the risk of disease. Planting too close together, on the other hand, can leave too much open space, letting weeds take over. The proper spacing depends on the type of herb and its mature size; therefore, be careful to look up this information for each plant.

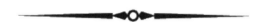

The journey doesn't stop once your herbs are in the ground or pot. The real test of your green thumb begins now. You've become the caretaker for these plants, and your attention and effort will be the keys to their growth and health. With some fundamental tips, you'll be able to nurture your plants with ease.

Watering Wisely

Watering is a critical aspect of herb care, but it's not as simple as it seems. The goal is to strike a balance because both overwatering and underwatering can harm your plants. Most herbs prefer the soil to be slightly dry before being watered again. When you water, water deeply, encouraging the roots to grow downwards.

A good rule of thumb is to check the top inch of soil. If it's dry, it's time to water. If it's still moist, wait for another day or two. Container plants will likely need more frequent watering as they dry out faster.

Feed Your Plants

Feeding your herbs is a way of replenishing and adding nutrients to the soil. Most herbs are not heavy feeders but will benefit from an occasional boost. A top dressing of compost or a dose of organic, slow-release fertilizer in the spring can provide a steady supply of nutrients throughout the growing season.

Weeding Regularly

Weeds compete with your herbs for resources, so regular weeding is necessary. Plus, a well-kept garden is much more pleasing to the eye! Mulching around your plants can help suppress weeds and also conserve soil moisture.

Pruning and Harvesting

Pruning helps maintain the shape and size of your plants and encourages denser growth. Regular harvesting of leaves and flowers also works as a sort of pruning, promoting further production.

For most herbs, it's best to harvest in the morning after the dew has dried but before the sun gets too hot. This is when the essential oils, which give herbs their aroma and flavor, are at their peak.

Watching for Pests and Diseases

Inspect your plants regularly for any signs of pests or diseases. Some common pests in the herb garden include aphids, slugs, and whiteflies. If you spot any, a blast of water from the hose or an application of insecticidal soap can help keep them in check. Early detection of problems can mean the difference between a little setback and a severe loss.

As for diseases, good cultural practices can prevent most issues. This includes avoiding overhead watering, which can encourage fungal diseases, and ensuring your plants have good air circulation.

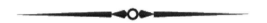

Bear in mind that every garden is unique, and what works for one may not work for another. It's all about observing, learning, and adapting to the specific needs of your plants and the conditions of your garden. Over time, you'll develop a routine that works best for you and your herbs. Most importantly, enjoy the process! Gardening is as much about the journey as it is about the destination.

Harvesting and Preserving Herbs

Harvesting and preserving herbs is a rewarding culmination of your careful planting and nurturing efforts. It is not just about plucking leaves off the plant; it's a thoughtful process that can significantly impact the potency and flavor of your herbs.

When it comes to harvesting, timing is fundamental. For most herbs, the best time to harvest is in the morning after the dew has evaporated but before the sun gets too hot. This is when the plant's essential oils are at their peak, giving you the most flavor and aromatic potency.

When you harvest, do so with care. Use sharp, clean scissors or pruners to make clean cuts. Generally, taking only about one-third of the plant at a time would be best, allowing it to recover and continue growing. However, some fast-growing herbs like mint and basil can handle more aggressive harvesting.

Preserving your herbs allows you to enjoy their flavors and health benefits long after the growing season has ended. There are several methods to preserve herbs, but the most common are drying and freezing.

Drying is a traditional method that works best with herbs like rosemary, thyme, and oregano. You can air-dry herbs by bundling them and hanging them upside down in a well-ventilated, dark location. Alternatively, you can use a dehydrator or an oven set to a low temperature for quicker results. Once the herbs are completely dry, remove the leaves from the stems and store them in an airtight container.

Freezing is another excellent way to preserve herbs, particularly those with high moisture content, like basil, parsley, and cilantro. To freeze herbs, you can either blanch them briefly in boiling water and then transfer them to ice water before freezing or freeze them in oil or ice cube trays. Once the cubes are frozen, transfer them to a freezer bag or container for long-term storage.

Let's keep in mind that preserved herbs can't quite match the taste of fresh ones, but they sure know how to bring the essence of the growing season to your dishes. With your own stash of homegrown and carefully preserved herbs, you can sprinkle a burst of flavor onto your meals all year long.

Troubleshooting Your Medicinal Herb Garden

1. Seed Germination Failure

One of the most common issues novices face is seeds fail to germinate. This could be due to many factors: old or poor-quality seeds, incorrect temperature, improper soil moisture, or poor lighting. To fix this, get seeds from a reliable source and double-check the germination rate listed on the packaging. Plant them at the recommended depth and keep the soil moist but not wet. Check that they are in the proper temperature range and have enough light.

2. Poor Growth

If your herbs grow slowly or seem stunted, they might lack nutrients, light, or space. Regularly feed them with a balanced organic fertilizer, ensuring they get enough light (6-8 hours for most herbs), and space them properly so they're not competing for resources.

3. Yellowing Leaves

Yellow leaves can be a sign of overwatering, poor drainage, or nutrient deficiency. If the soil is constantly wet, consider reducing the watering frequency and ensure the pot or bed has good drainage. If it's a nutrient deficiency, typically nitrogen, supplementing with an appropriate fertilizer should help.

4. Pest Infestations

Aphids, mites, and slugs are common in herb gardens. Regularly inspect your plants for signs of damage. You can remove pests manually or use natural deterrents like neem oil or insecticidal soaps. Encouraging beneficial insects, such as ladybugs and lacewings, can also help control pests.

- Disease: Fungi, bacteria, and viruses can all cause plant diseases. Prevention is key: keep your garden clean, don't overcrowd plants, and water in the morning so leaves can dry out during the day. If a plant does get diseased, remove and dispose of it away from the garden to prevent spreading.

- Wilting: Overwatering, underwatering, or a root disease could cause wilting. If the soil is too dry, water more frequently. If it's too wet, let it dry out before watering again. If the problem persists, it could be a root disease, which may require removing the plant.

- Bolting: It occurs when a plant goes to seed too soon, usually due to high temperatures or lengthy daylight hours. If you want to prevent this, provide shade during the warmest part of the day and harvest your herbs on a regular basis to encourage new leaf growth.

- Poor Flavor: If your herbs lack flavor, they might get too much fertilizer or water. Both can dilute the concentration of the oils that give herbs their taste and aroma. Reduce watering and feeding and see the difference.

- Leggy Plants: If plants reach toward the light, they become leggy (tall with sparse foliage). This is common in congested gardens or indoor gardens with little natural light. Make sure that your herbs are given at least 6-8 hours of light per day. You may need to supplement with grow lights if you're growing indoors.

- Frost Damage: If you live in a region with frost, delicate herbs could get damaged. Bring potted herbs indoors before the first frost to avoid this. Consider using row covers or cloches to protect them if they're in the ground. If your herbs are frost damaged, trim the affected areas in the spring to make room for fresh growth.

When it comes to gardening, patience, and observation are key. Pay attention to your plants and their needs, and don't be discouraged by setbacks. With time and experience, you will become more adept at recognizing and solving problems in your medicinal herb garden.

Chapter Three

Foraging: A Journey to Nature's Pharmacy

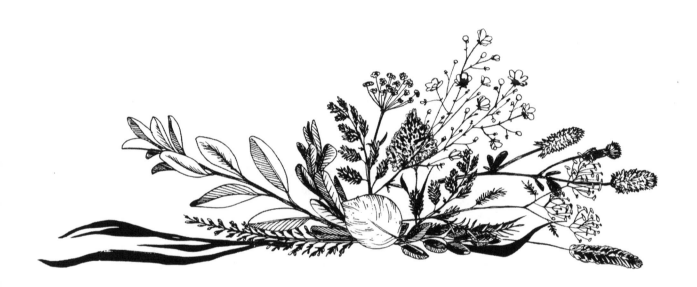

Ever since the dawn of time, our ancestors have been deeply connected to the natural world around them. Relying on nature for sustenance and medicine, they forged a path of survival that was rooted in the land itself. In the spirit of our forebearers, let's embark on a journey that will reconnect us with the wisdom of nature - the art and science of foraging.

At its core, foraging is the practice of collecting food and medicinal plants directly from their natural, wild habitats. It involves not only a deep knowledge of the plants and their uses but also the patience to observe nature, understanding the delicate balance between harvesting what is needed and ensuring the plant's survival for future generations.

The world of foraging opens the door to a myriad of benefits. At the very heart of it, foraging is an immersive experience, a walkabout in the wilderness that beckons us to breathe in the aroma of the earth and observe the subtle shift in the seasons. It instills a sense of mindfulness and helps us foster a deep connection with nature, the Earth, and its rhythmic cycles.

The tangible benefits of foraging are manifold:

- Enhanced Nutrition: Wild foods are often more nutrient-dense than their cultivated counterparts.

- Economic Savings: Foraging for edible and medicinal plants can help offset grocery costs.

- Physical Exercise: The act of foraging can be a great way to stay active and fit.

- Mental Well-being: Connecting with nature can reduce stress and improve mental health.

- Educational: Foraging encourages continuous learning about nature and plant species.

- Sustainability: It promotes self-reliance and lessens reliance on industrial agriculture.

However, foraging is not without its challenges. The forager's path is one of patience and persistence, filled with the joy of discovery but also the necessity of meticulous identification and mindful harvesting. Understanding the ecology of the area, knowing which plants are safe to consume or use medicinally, and respecting local regulations are all vital components of responsible foraging. It is a skill that demands diligence, learning, and a profound respect for Mother Nature.

Foraging and herbal remedies are intrinsically entwined. Most of our traditional herbal remedies were, in fact, born from the practice of foraging. As we walk in the footsteps of the ancients, we discover plants with remarkable healing properties that have been used for centuries. From the humble dandelion, a powerhouse of vitamins and minerals, to the soothing effects of wild chamomile, nature's pharmacy awaits us.

As a child, I would walk with my grandmother through the woodland trails behind our house. She had an intimate knowledge of the landscape and could spot a wild herb from a distance. I remember her fingers, weathered by time yet nimble, carefully picking the leaves and flowers, always leaving enough for the plant to thrive. She would whisper a quiet thank you to the plant, a simple yet powerful acknowledgement of the gift we were receiving. This is the essence of foraging - a practice that binds us to our roots, reminding us of the healing power of nature, and encouraging us to live sustainably and harmoniously within our environment.

So, let's lace up our hiking boots and pack our foraging bags, for there are fields to explore, plants to discover, and herbal remedies to create.

Ethics of Foraging

In the grand theatre of nature, every creature, plant, and microorganism plays a vital role. They contribute to the ecological balance, each species intertwined in a delicate, harmonious dance of life. As we step into the world of foraging, it is paramount to remember that we are visitors in this theatre, and our actions can have significant consequences. Therefore, the cornerstone of foraging lies not just in the knowledge of plants and their uses but in the principles of ethical foraging that guide us towards sustainable practices.

One of the key tenets of ethical foraging is sustainability. Our role is not to deplete, but to participate in nature's rhythm, ensuring the continued flourishing of the plant species we harvest. Sustainability in foraging goes beyond the immediate act of picking a plant - it extends to understanding the life cycle of each species, the optimal time for harvest, and the best way to do it, ensuring the plant's regeneration.

Consider, for example, the case of the wild leek, also known as ramps. These plants are a delicacy among foragers, but their popularity has led to overharvesting, endangering their survival in certain areas. Ramps take several years to mature and produce seeds, and pulling up the entire plant (a common practice among inexperienced foragers) prevents it from reproducing. Sustainable foraging would involve only taking a few leaves from each plant, leaving the bulb in the ground to ensure future growth.

The second ethical consideration is about respect, a deeply ingrained sense of reverence towards the natural world. As my grandfather used to say, "Take only what you need, and leave the rest for nature and others to enjoy." This philosophy emphasizes that nature is a shared space, a common heritage, and we need to respect the needs of other creatures and humans who also rely on these resources.

There's an interesting example from the world of mushrooms. Certain fungi have symbiotic relationships with trees, aiding in nutrient exchange. Overharvesting these mushrooms can disrupt this relationship, affecting the health of the entire forest. An ethical forager recognizes this interdependence and ensures that their actions don't disrupt these natural partnerships.

Lastly, understanding and abiding by local laws and regulations is essential. Not all areas are open to foraging, and certain plant species may be protected due to their ecological importance or threatened status. Did you know, for instance, that in some parts of the United States, it is illegal to forage ginseng, a plant highly prized for its medicinal properties, due to its endangered status? Ignorance of these laws not only harms the environment but can also lead to legal repercussions.

In conclusion, ethical foraging is about maintaining a harmonious relationship with nature. It is about ensuring sustainability, showing respect, and adhering to the laws that protect our precious ecosystems. As we venture into the wild with basket in hand, let's remember to tread lightly, for we are the stewards of the land, and our actions today will determine the health of our Earth tomorrow.

Safety and Risk Management

Embarking on the path of foraging can feel like stepping into a real-life treasure hunt. The thrill of discovery, the joy of connecting with nature, and the gratification of self-reliance are profoundly rewarding. Yet, this journey is not without its hazards. An essential aspect of foraging is understanding the potential risks and adopting strategies to ensure your safety and the integrity of the plants you collect. Let's delve into some of these critical aspects.

Arguably the most crucial safety aspect in foraging is correct plant identification. The natural world is replete with a variety of plant species, some of which closely resemble one another. While one might be a bountiful source of nutrition or medicine, its look-alike could be harmful or even lethal. For instance, the harmless Wild Carrot and the toxic Water Hemlock share a striking resemblance. Misidentification of these could lead to severe poisoning. To avoid this risk, it's imperative to familiarize yourself with the plants in your region, preferably under the guidance of an experienced forager or botanist. Always follow the forager's golden rule: Never consume a plant unless you're 100% certain of its identification.

The second factor to consider is the risk of contamination. Plants, being the incredible bio-factories they are, absorb nutrients from the soil but can also take in harmful substances. Foraging near roads, industrial areas, or polluted waterways increases the risk of collecting plants contaminated with heavy metals, chemicals, or other toxins. Even a wonderfully nutrient-rich plant like stinging nettle can become a health hazard if it's grown in contaminated soil. As a forager, it's crucial to understand the history and health of the area where you plan to forage.

Lastly, let's not forget that when we step into the wilderness, we step into the home of countless other creatures. Foraging involves navigating these shared spaces responsibly and safely. Depending on your location, you may encounter animals or insects that pose a threat. In North America, for example, you might stumble upon a patch of blackberries, only to find it's already claimed by a bear! Knowing how to react in such situations is vital. Additionally, insects like ticks and mosquitoes can be a nuisance and a health risk. Wearing appropriate clothing, using natural repellents, and checking for ticks after your foraging adventure can help mitigate these risks.

Foraging Tools and Techniques

Basic Tools for Foraging

Setting foot on the foraging path can be an exhilarating experience. The fresh air, the rustle of leaves underfoot, and the anticipation of discovering nature's bounty - all these elements combined paint a serene and vibrant picture. Yet, to make the most of this adventure and to ensure the longevity of the natural habitats we explore, it's essential to equip ourselves with the right tools. These not only make the process easier but also play a crucial role in minimizing damage to the plants and the surrounding ecosystem.

Firstly, we need to talk about a forager's best friend - a sturdy, reliable bag or basket. From carrying your finds to doubling up as an impromptu seat, this item is an absolute must. Opt for a basket woven from natural materials or a durable fabric bag with good weight distribution, like a backpack. Avoid plastic bags as they can cause delicate plants to wilt quickly due to lack of air circulation.

Next on our list of essentials is a good quality pair of gloves. Whether you're reaching into thorny bushes, handling plants that can cause skin irritations, or digging in the dirt, a pair of gloves can protect your hands from potential harm. Choose gloves that are tough yet offer enough flexibility for intricate tasks, such as picking small berries or delicate leaves.

A reliable, sharp knife is another essential tool in a forager's kit. From cutting through tough stems to digging up roots, a knife comes in handy in many situations. Opt for a foldable, pocket-sized knife with a sturdy handle and a sharp blade. Remember, using a dull knife can lead to accidental slips, so keep your blade sharp and handle it with care.

Hand trowels or hori-hori (a Japanese gardening knife) are invaluable when it comes to digging up roots or bulbs. They allow you to dig without causing extensive damage to the surrounding vegetation. If you decide to carry one, make sure it's made from sturdy, rust-resistant material and is easy to clean.

Last but not least, consider carrying a field guide or a plant identification app. These resources can assist you in identifying plants correctly, thereby increasing your safety and enhancing your understanding of the flora around you. Opt for guides or apps specific to your region for the most accurate information.

While these tools form the basics of a forager's kit, remember that the most important tool you possess is your awareness and respect for nature. By being conscious of our actions and equipped with the right tools, we can ensure that our foraging adventures are fruitful and respectful, allowing us to savor the gifts of nature while preserving its beauty for generations to come.

Foraging Techniques

While having the right tools for foraging is essential, understanding how to use them effectively and responsibly is equally important. Proper foraging techniques ensure not only the sustainability of plant populations but also the quality of the bounty you collect. So, let's dive into some of these methods.

When it comes to gathering leaves, flowers, or fruits from plants, the "snap and twist" technique is often used. This involves gently gripping the stem and twisting it until it snaps. By using this method, you avoid tearing the plant unnecessarily, which could leave it vulnerable to diseases or pests. A small knife can also be useful for cleanly cutting stems and minimizing damage.

For plants where you're interested in the root, digging requires a bit more care. The key is to disturb the surrounding soil as little as possible. With the help of a hand trowel or hori-hori, carefully dig around the plant, ensuring you give yourself enough space to avoid damaging the root. Once the plant is free, gently shake off the excess soil, ensuring the least amount of impact on the environment.

When foraging for berries, remember that they do not all ripen at the same time. Practice selective picking, only choosing the berries that are ripe and leaving the others to mature. This approach not only gives you the sweetest fruits but also ensures a longer harvesting period.

It's also essential to note that some plants propagate through their leaves or stems. In these cases, make sure you leave a significant part of the plant behind. This practice allows the plant to recover quickly and continue growing. For example, when foraging for wild onions, leaving the bottom part of the bulb in the ground will enable the plant to regrow.

Another critical aspect to keep in mind is the concept of moderation. Even if a plant is abundant, resist the temptation to harvest more than you need. A good rule of thumb to follow is the "Rule of Thirds" - only take a third of what's available, leave a third for nature, and a third for other foragers.

Timing in Foraging

As a forager, knowing the best time to harvest is as vital as knowing what to harvest and how. Different plants, even different parts of the same plant, have their unique 'prime times' when their flavors, nutritional content, or medicinal properties are at their peak. Recognizing these windows can greatly enhance the quality of your forage and also contribute to sustainable harvesting.

For most herbs and leafy greens, the best time to harvest is just before the plant begins to flower. At this stage, the plant has reached its peak vigor, and the leaves are typically the most flavorful and nutrient-dense. Harvesting in the morning, after the dew has dried but before the sun is at its peak, is also recommended. During this time, the plant's essential oils are the most concentrated, making it ideal for those interested in their medicinal properties.

When it comes to harvesting flowers, timing can be quite specific. Many blossoms, such as chamomile or calendula, should ideally be picked just after they've fully opened. As for fruiting plants, it's best to wait until the fruit is fully ripe. However, be sure to harvest before the fruits start to decay or before birds and insects have had their share.

Roots and bulbs, such as ginseng or wild leeks, have a different harvesting timeline. The best time to collect these is usually in late fall or early spring when the plant's energy is concentrated in the roots, and the above-ground parts are dormant. But remember, over-harvesting of roots can severely impact plant populations, so be sure to use sustainable practices, like only taking a small amount from each cluster and replanting parts of the root when possible.

Lastly, timing isn't only about seasons or the time of day. It's also about understanding and respecting the natural cycles of the plant populations. After a particularly harsh winter or drought, it may be best to let the plant community recover for a season before foraging. Likewise, if a certain species seems less abundant than usual, it might be time to seek out other resources and give that plant a chance to rebound.

Commonly Foraged Medicinal Plants

In the verdant wilds of North America, an array of medicinal plants wait to be discovered. While the detailed information on each plant, including its medicinal uses, harvesting tips, and more, can be found in the subsequent chapters of this book, let's focus here on a brief overview of some of the commonly found medicinal plants. Please remember, accurate plant identification is crucial, so always cross-reference with a reliable field guide or app.

- Stinging Nettle (Urtica dioica): Found in rich, moist soil near streams or in open woods, this plant is easily recognizable by its tiny, hair-like stingers. Wear gloves to avoid the stinging sensation when harvesting.

- Dandelion (Taraxacum officinale): This common 'weed' thrives in a variety of conditions, including lawns, meadows, and even sidewalk cracks. Its entire plant can be harvested, from root to flower.

- Plantain (Plantago major): Often found growing in lawns or disturbed soils, plantain has distinctive ribbed leaves. It's best to forage the young leaves before the plant flowers.

- Yarrow (Achillea millefolium): Yarrow prefers sunny open fields and roadsides with well-drained soil. The flowers, which bloom from late spring to fall, are usually harvested.

- Burdock (Arctium lappa): Commonly found along roadsides, fields, or waste places, burdock is usually harvested for its roots in the fall of its first year or the spring of its second year.

- Elderberry (Sambucus nigra): This plant loves moist areas near streams or rivers and is usually harvested for its berries in late summer to fall.

- Wild Ginger (Asarum canadense): Found in rich, moist, deciduous forests, wild ginger's roots are usually harvested in the fall.

- Mullein (Verbascum thapsus): Commonly found in open, sunny areas with well-drained soil, its leaves are best harvested in its first year, and flowers are collected in its second year.

- Red Clover (Trifolium pratense): This plant prefers fields and pastures, and it's the flowers that are commonly harvested in summer.

- Chickweed (Stellaria media): Thriving in cool, moist, shady areas, its leaves and stems are best harvested in the spring before it flowers.

An helpful app

As just mentioned, proper plant identification is paramount to ensure a safe and successful foraging experience. One app that can be tremendously helpful for this purpose is PlantNet Plant Identification.

PlantNet is a plant identification app designed to help you identify plants based on photographs. By simply taking a picture with your smartphone, you can get instant suggestions about the plant's identity. It uses a database of several million referenced plant images to make identifications.

The app is collaborative and uses a powerful image recognition technology combined with data provided by botanists from around the world. It's a valuable tool not only for plant identification but also for those interested in contributing to a large-scale scientific database of flora across the globe.

It's important to note that while PlantNet is a great aid for plant identification, it's not infallible. It's essential to cross-check the information it provides, particularly when you're dealing with plants that have lookalikes. Also, remember that PlantNet's effectiveness can depend on the quality and clarity of the image you provide.

So while out in the field, snap clear photos, use PlantNet for preliminary identification, and then cross-verify with a trusted field guide or local expert, especially when foraging for medicinal plants. Safety first!

Preservation and Storage of Foraged Herbs

Cleaning Harvested Herbs

After returning from a successful foraging expedition, with your basket brimming with nature's gifts, the next crucial step is cleaning your harvest. This process, though seemingly simple, plays a pivotal role in maintaining the potency, flavor, and overall quality of the herbs you've collected.

Before you start the cleaning process, it's important to have a workspace that is clean and free from contaminants. A clean cutting board, fresh water, and clean, dry towels will be the essentials needed.

Begin by sorting through your harvested herbs. Separate them into groups by species to make the cleaning process more organized. This also gives you a chance to do one final check for correct identification of each plant. Remember, accuracy is paramount when dealing with medicinal herbs.

Start the cleaning process by gently shaking each herb to remove any loose soil or debris. Do this outside if possible to keep your indoor workspace clean. If the plant has larger leaves, like plantain or burdock, you can brush off the dirt using your fingers or a soft brush. For smaller, delicate leaves or flowers, take care not to damage them in the process.

Next, fill a large bowl or basin with cold water. Immerse the herbs in the water, giving them a gentle swirl. This helps to dislodge any remaining dirt. Depending on how dirty they are, you may need to repeat this process a couple of times, always with fresh water.

Remember, it's best to avoid washing delicate herbs like yarrow or red clover until you're ready to use them, as excess water can make them wilt quickly. For these, just a gentle shake to remove any dirt or insects should suffice.

Once cleaned, gently pat the herbs dry using a clean towel. Try not to rub the herbs as this can bruise them and lead to loss of essential oils. For herbs with a lot of crevices or multiple small leaves, consider using a salad spinner to help remove excess water without damaging the plant.

Drying and Storing Herbs

Once you've cleaned your herbs, the next step is preservation. While there are several methods available, drying is one of the most traditional and effective ways to maintain the medicinal properties of the herbs for extended periods.

Drying herbs is a delicate balance - you need to remove moisture quickly to prevent decay but do it slowly enough to retain the essential oils and medicinal properties. Here are some techniques to achieve this:

- Air Drying: This is the simplest method and works well with many herbs. Bundle your herbs loosely and hang them upside down in a dry, well-ventilated area out of direct sunlight. Herbs with high moisture content like plantain or burdock may mold if not dried quickly enough, so consider removing the leaves from the stems and laying them out flat to dry.

- Dehydrator: If you have access to a dehydrator, it can speed up the drying process and can be particularly useful for herbs with a high moisture content. Remember to set the dehydrator at the lowest setting (usually around 95°F or 35°C) to preserve the medicinal properties.

- Oven Drying: If you don't have a dehydrator, an oven set at the lowest temperature with the door slightly open can serve a similar function. Arrange the herbs on a baking sheet in a single layer for even drying. This method requires careful monitoring to prevent overheating, which can degrade the herbs' medicinal qualities.

Once the herbs are completely dry, they should crumble easily, and the stems should snap. Remember, over-dried herbs can lose their potency, so aim for just the right level of dryness.

After drying, store your herbs in an airtight container like a glass jar, out of direct sunlight. Label your jars with the name of the herb and the date of preservation. Keep them in a cool, dry place. Properly stored, most dried herbs can maintain their potency for up to a year.

Using Freshly Foraged Herbs

While drying and storing herbs is a fantastic way to enjoy the benefits of your foraging efforts all year round, there's also something incredibly rewarding about using freshly foraged herbs. Their vibrant color, aroma, and full potency make them a remarkable addition to a variety of preparations and recipes. Here are a few ways to put your fresh herbs to use:

- Herbal Teas: Perhaps one of the simplest and most satisfying ways to enjoy fresh herbs is by making a herbal tea, or infusion. Simply steep a handful of herbs in hot water for about 10-15 minutes, strain, and enjoy. From the soothing effects of chamomile to the invigorating properties of nettle, the possibilities are endless.

- Salves and Ointments: Freshly harvested herbs can be used to create healing salves and ointments. These typically involve infusing the herbs in a carrier oil, such as olive oil, and then combining this with beeswax to form a soothing topical application.

- Fresh in Cooking: Many medicinal herbs can also serve as culinary herbs. Fresh dandelion leaves can be used in salads, nettle can be cooked and used much like spinach, and wild garlic can bring a wonderful flavor to soups and stir-fries.

- Herbal Baths: This may sound decadent, but a herbal bath can be a wonderful way to enjoy the soothing properties of your foraged finds. Tie a bunch of herbs in a piece of muslin or cheesecloth, hang it under the hot tap as you run your bath, and let the beneficial properties of the herbs infuse the water.

- Tinctures: A tincture is a concentrated herbal extract. It's created by soaking herbs in a high-proof alcohol which extracts the beneficial compounds. Tinctures are typically used in small doses and can have a longer shelf life than other herbal preparations.

Building a Foraging Community

Foraging for medicinal herbs is not just a solitary pursuit. It can be a wonderfully social activity that connects people, not only to nature but also to each other. There is something inherently communal about venturing into the wilds as a group, exploring, discovering, and learning together.

The Benefits of Foraging in Groups

Firstly, there's the practical aspect: safety. Foraging in groups can provide an additional level of safety, particularly when exploring unfamiliar terrains or when foraging for less well-known plants. More pairs of eyes can help spot potential hazards, and there's reassurance in knowing that if anything were to go wrong, you're not alone.

Additionally, foraging in groups presents excellent learning opportunities. Those with more experience can share their knowledge, helping newcomers learn to identify different plants, understand where and when to harvest them, and how to prepare them for use. Novices, on the other hand, may offer fresh perspectives and spark new insights. It's a synergistic relationship that enriches everyone involved.

Finally, the social connection that forms when foraging in groups is something quite special. The shared experience of being in nature, of learning and discovering together, can foster deep bonds of friendship. For many, these connections, forged under the open sky and amidst the rustling leaves, become as invaluable as the plants they gather.

Connecting with Local Foraging Communities

To connect with local foraging communities, start by looking for clubs or groups in your area that are dedicated to foraging, herbalism, or related fields. Local nature centers or botanical gardens often run workshops or guided walks that can serve as an excellent introduction to the local foraging scene. Online platforms like Meetup or Facebook can also be useful to find relevant groups.

Organizing Foraging Trips

If you're thinking about organizing a foraging trip, there are a few things to consider. First, plan your location based on the time of year and the plants you're hoping to find. Always ensure that foraging is permitted in the area you've chosen. Plan your trip so that everyone knows where to meet, what to bring, and what the goals of the trip are.

Before setting out, ensure everyone knows the guidelines of ethical foraging, and set a good example by following these principles yourself. It's also important to keep safety in mind: everyone should be aware of potential hazards and know what to do in case of an emergency.

The act of foraging is an ancient tradition that has brought people together for millennia. In today's fast-paced, technology-driven world, forming a foraging community can help us reconnect with nature, with our ancestors, and with each other. Happy foraging!

BOOK VII

NATURAL HEALING TECHNIQUES

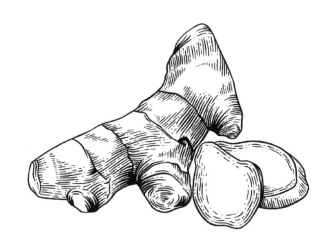

AMBER WHITMORE

Introduction

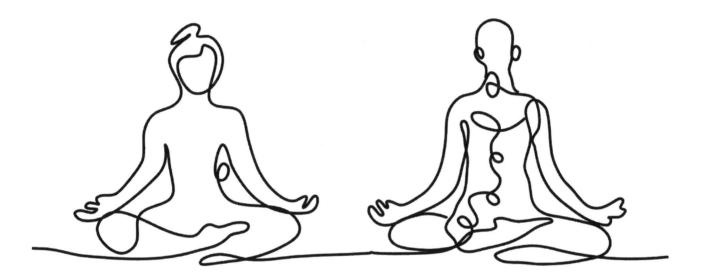

Given their widespread popularity, conversations around natural medicine often steer straight toward herbal remedies. However, it is particularly important to cast a wider net and acknowledge the rich diversity of different natural healing approaches that deserve to be recognized. This book is designed as a comprehensive guide for beginners, aiming to shed light on the myriad of other holistic healing modalities that beautifully complement the herbal knowledge we've previously unearthed.

We will delve into the ancient practices of Yoga and Meditation, which have been used for centuries to promote physical and mental wellness. We will explore the intriguing world of Acupressure and Acupuncture, traditional Chinese medicine techniques known for balancing the body's energy flow. Next, we will immerse ourselves in the aromatic world of Aromatherapy and Essential Oils, discussing how these potent extracts can influence our mood and well-being.

Our journey will then take us to the realm of Homeopathy, a form of alternative medicine that employs heavily diluted substances to trigger the body's natural healing response.

The following pages aim to provide a panoramic view of natural healing, broadening our understanding of the multitude of ways in which we can harness the natural world for our health and wellness. As we explore each healing technique, remember that the health journey is personal, and what works for one may not work for another.

Chapter One

Yoga and Meditation

The origins of Yoga can be traced back to the ancient civilizations of India, where this practice has a rich history dating back over 5,000 years. Over centuries, Yoga evolved, incorporating physical postures (asanas), breath control (pranayama), and meditation (dhyana) to promote physical strength, mental clarity, and spiritual growth.

Meditation has ancient origins, appearing in various forms across many cultures. However, it found its most profound and well-documented development in the Buddhist traditions of East Asia. Meditation was considered a way to calm the mind, cultivate inner peace, and ultimately achieve enlightenment.

In today's modern world, both Yoga and Meditation have been adopted globally, transcending their religious origins. They are revered for spiritual growth and their remarkable benefits to physical and mental well-being.

Yoga is based on the idea of creating balance in the body by developing both strength and flexibility. This is achieved through poses or postures, each with specific physical benefits. Meditation, on the other hand, is about turning inward. It is a practice of quieting the mind and fostering deep inner peace. Meditation involves focusing the mind—often on the breath, a word, or a phrase—and gently bringing it back when it wanders. This process helps to develop a greater awareness of the present moment.

Incredibly, Yoga and Meditation share the same goal: to achieve a state of mindfulness in which we are totally present and engaged. As we continue to investigate these methods, keep an open mind, patience, and a spirit of curiosity in mind. Who knows what wonderful discoveries you could make along the way regarding your potential for growth and healing?

The Science Behind Yoga and Meditation

Every time we attend these practices, it is as if we are unmasking an invisible dance in our bodies. From the tips of our fingers to the depths of our minds, these ancient disciplines touch every aspect of our being, creating a symphony of beneficial changes.

Starting with Yoga, each pose or asana engages specific muscles, enhancing strength, flexibility, and balance. These physical changes ripple outwards, affecting our cardiovascular system by improving circulation and reducing heart rate. Yoga also supports our respiratory system: our lung capacity can increase as we consciously control our breathing during practice.

Yoga's effects seep into our nervous system, too. By helping to lower the body's stress response, it can promote a sense of relaxation and ease. This calming effect is partly why many people find their sleep quality improves with regular yoga practice.

Turning our gaze to Meditation, we find this practice primarily impacts our brain and nervous system. It cultivates a state of relaxation that can lower blood pressure, reduce anxiety, and enhance mood. Meditators often report feeling less stressed and more focused. Fascinatingly, studies have shown that regular meditation can alter the brain's structure, increasing density in areas linked to self-awareness, empathy, and stress regulation.

Scientific study affirms the healing benefits of these practices. According to studies on neuroimaging, mindfulness meditation can remodel the brain's gray matter, improving memory, self-awareness, empathy, stress control, and creativity while lowering anxiety and increasing attention. In recently published research, yoga can increase mobility in older adults while decreasing Post Traumatic Stress Disorder symptoms.

Different Types of Yoga

Yoga's versatility shines through in the various styles that have developed over time, each with its unique approach and benefits. Let's take a closer look at four popular types of yoga that cater to different needs and preferences:

Hatha Yoga

Let's begin our tour of yoga styles with Hatha Yoga, a particularly beginner-friendly style. 'Hatha' is a composite of 'Ha,' which means sun, and 'Tha,' which means moon. This style aims to balance these two energies within us. Hatha Yoga focuses on slow and gentle movements, allowing plenty of time to explore each pose and understand the alignment. It's a beautiful style for promoting flexibility and calming the mind.

Vinyasa Yoga

Next, we venture into Vinyasa Yoga, a style characterized by its fluid, movement-intensive practice. 'Vinyasa' translates to 'arranging something in a special way,' like yoga poses. This style often synchronizes breath with movement, creating a dynamic, flowing sequence of poses that feels almost like a dance. Vinyasa might be just the ticket for a more physically engaging yoga style.

Restorative Yoga

Restorative Yoga is a terrific approach to de-stress and rejuvenate, as well as to cultivate a deep sense of inner serenity. Restorative Yoga, as the name implies, is all about relaxation and restoration. Props such as blankets, bolsters, and yoga blocks are used to fully support the body in each pose, helping you to relax deeply and let go.

Kundalini Yoga

Finally, we arrive at Kundalini Yoga, a style that blends physical postures, breathing techniques, meditation, and the chanting of mantras. Kundalini Yoga aims to awaken the energy at the base of the spine and draw it upward through each of the seven chakras. This style can offer a profoundly transformative experience, fostering emotional release and heightening self-awareness.

Yoga Postures (Asanas)

Yoga poses, or asanas, are designed to target specific areas of the body and offer a range of therapeutic benefits. Here are a few examples of common postures and their effects:

- Child's Pose (Balasana): Gently stretches the back, hips, and thighs, promoting relaxation and stress relief.

- Downward-Facing Dog (Adho Mukha Svanasana): Stretches the hamstrings, calves, and shoulders while strengthening the arms and legs. It also helps to alleviate mild back pain.

- Tree Pose (Vrksasana): Improves balance, focus, and concentration while strengthening the legs and core muscles.

- Warrior II (Virabhadrasana II): Strengthens and stretches the legs, hips, and shoulders while fostering determination and inner strength.

While yoga is generally considered safe, it's always wise to keep a few guidelines in mind to ensure a beneficial and injury-free practice:

1. Consult a doctor before starting, especially if you have any pre-existing medical conditions or concerns.

2. Begin with a qualified yoga instructor to learn proper alignment and technique.

3. Listen to your body, and never push yourself into pain or discomfort.

4. Modify postures to accommodate your body's unique needs and limitations.

5. Use props like blocks, straps, or bolsters to support your practice.

6. Remember to breathe deeply and evenly throughout the session.

7. Be consistent in your practice, but also be patient with yourself as you progress.

Different Types of Meditation

Just as there are many styles of yoga, there are also various forms of meditation, each with its unique focus and benefits. Let's explore three common types of meditation:

Mindfulness Meditation

Origin: Rooted in Buddhist traditions, popularized in the West by Jon Kabat-Zinn

Characteristics: Involves paying attention to present-moment experiences with openness and curiosity

Benefits:

1. Fosters a deeper awareness of the present moment

2. Reduces stress and enhances mental clarity

3. Cultivates a non-judgmental attitude toward oneself and others

Transcendental Meditation

Origin: Introduced by Maharishi Mahesh Yogi in the 1950s

Characteristics: Involves repeating a personal mantra in a specific way

Benefits:

1. Promotes deep relaxation and stress relief

2. Enhances self-awareness and fosters a sense of peace

3. May improve cardiovascular health

Loving-Kindness Meditation (Metta Meditation)

Origin: Based on Buddhist teachings, particularly the practice of metta

Characteristics: Involves cultivating feelings of love, kindness, and goodwill toward oneself and others

Benefits:

1. Fosters positive emotions toward oneself and others

2. Reduces negative emotions like anger and frustration

3. Can improve interpersonal relationships

Techniques for Effective Meditation

Starting a meditation practice can seem daunting, but remember that it's not about achieving a particular state but rather about familiarizing yourself with the workings of your mind. Here are some steps to help you get started:

1. Find a quiet, comfortable space where you won't be disturbed.

2. Sit comfortably. You can sit on a cushion on the floor or a chair if that's more comfortable. The key is to keep your back straight to allow for deep, easy breaths.

3. Choose your focus, which could be your breath, a word, a phrase, or even the sensations in your body.

4. Close your eyes and start to bring your attention to your chosen focus.

5. When your mind wanders, gently guide it back without judgment.

6. Start with short, five-minute sessions, and gradually increase the time as you become more comfortable with the practice.

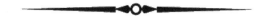

Breath plays a central role in most forms of meditation. It serves as an anchor, keeping you grounded in the present moment. Noticing the coolness of the inhale, the brief pause between breaths, and the warmth of the exhale can bring a profound sense of calm and focus. When you focus on your breath, you tune into a basic and life-sustaining process that often goes unnoticed.

Furthermore, breath awareness can aid with emotional regulation. Slow, deep breaths can activate the relaxation response in the body, lowering tension and encouraging peace of mind. The breath is a faithful companion on your journey toward greater awareness, regardless of what kind of meditation you choose to practice.

Integrating Yoga and Meditation into Daily Life

Imagine creating a personal oasis of tranquility, a refuge from the whirlwind of daily life where you can nourish your body, mind, and spirit. That's what designing a personal Yoga and Meditation routine can offer you.

The beauty of these practices is their adaptability to fit into your unique lifestyle. There's no one-size-fits-all approach here. Instead, it's about crafting a routine that resonates with your needs and circumstances.

So, how might you go about creating such a routine?

Start by establishing your schedule. Can you practice in the morning, midday, or evening? Perhaps you could begin your day with a few yoga poses to wake up your body and end it with a relaxing meditation to prepare for sleep.

Next, think about the space you have available. Can you create a dedicated area for your practice? It doesn't need to be large or extravagant; just a quiet corner where you can roll out a yoga mat or sit comfortably to meditate.

Now, think about what you want to focus on. Maybe you wish to build strength and flexibility or seek stress relief or a deeper sense of self-awareness. Choose yoga poses and meditation techniques that align with your goals.

For instance, if you want to start your day with energy and focus, you might choose a sequence of Sun Salutations in yoga and mindfulness meditation. On the other hand, if you're aiming for deep relaxation before bed, restorative yoga poses and a guided body scan meditation could be your go-to.

Remember, your routine can evolve as you do. Feel free to experiment and adjust as needed.

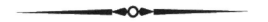

Just as a seed needs consistent watering to sprout and grow, your Yoga and Meditation practice requires regularity to yield its full benefits.

Consistency doesn't necessarily mean spending hours on the mat or meditation cushion each day. Instead, it's about maintaining regular practice, whether 15 minutes a day or an hour weekly.

Think about the rhythm of brushing your teeth or taking a daily shower. These activities are woven into your daily routine, often performed without much thought yet vital for your well-being. Similarly, consistent practice of Yoga and Meditation can become a natural and cherished part of your daily rhythm.

With regular practice, you'll likely notice gradual improvements in your flexibility and strength from yoga and enhanced focus and tranquility from meditation. However, the advantages go beyond the physical. You may also notice higher self-awareness, a stronger connection to your inner self, and an improved capacity to deal with life's twists and turns with compassion and perseverance over time.

Chapter Two

Acupressure and Acupuncture

Acupressure and Acupuncture are two closely related healing practices rooted in the ancient traditions of Chinese medicine. These therapeutic approaches, which date back more than 2000 years, are based on the notion of life energy, known as "Qi" (pronounced "chi"), flowing through the body.

Acupressure is a technique where pressure is applied to specific points on the body using the hands, fingers, or special devices to stimulate and balance the flow of Qi. Acupuncture, conversely, involves inserting fine needles into specific points on the body to achieve similar results.

Acupressure and acupuncture, while using different approaches, enhance health and wellness by balancing the body's energy flow. These practices have withstood the test of time and have been recognized as essential components of holistic health.

Basic Principles and Theories

Qi (Energy Flow)

Envision for a moment a flowing river. When unobstructed, the water moves freely, cascading over rocks and winding through the landscape. In Chinese medicine, this metaphor illustrates the concept of Qi (pronounced "chi"), the life force or vital energy that moves within us. This invisible energy is said to animate us and support our overall health and vitality.

Like the river, when Qi flows freely within us, we experience good health and well-being. However, if there are "blockages" or "stagnations" in this flow, much like a dam in the river, health problems can occur. These blockages can be released through practices like acupressure and acupuncture, allowing Qi to flow freely once again.

Meridians (Energy Channels)

Now, imagine the extensive network of roads and highways across a country, facilitating transport and connection. According to Chinese Medicine, the body has a similar network, but instead of roads, these are "meridians" or "energy channels." These meridians connect different body areas and act as pathways for Qi.

There are twelve primary meridians, each associated with a specific organ system and each with a set of acupoints. In a healthy body, energy travels smoothly through these meridians, like cars moving smoothly on well-maintained roads. If a roadblock occurs, traffic gets backed up. Similarly, in the body, disruptions or blockages in the meridians can lead to health issues.

Yin and Yang

Yin and Yang is a foundational philosophy in Chinese medicine that embodies the principle of dualism. Picture a sunny day at the beach: the sun (yang) provides heat and light, while the sea (yin) is cool and tranquil. Neither is superior to the other; instead, they are interdependent and complementary, each contributing to the harmony of the beach experience.

Similarly, Yin and Yang in the body represent opposite but complementary energies that need to balance each other. Yang is often associated with heat, action, and function, while Yin represents coolness, rest, and structure. The ultimate goal of practices like acupressure and acupuncture is to foster a harmonious balance between Yin and Yang, facilitating the smooth flow of Qi and promoting optimal health.

Differences between Acupressure and Acupuncture

1. Tools Used

Acupressure and acupuncture are two different techniques that use specific tools to achieve their respective goals. Acupressure involves applying pressure using fingers, hands, or specialized devices like acupressure mats or sticks. Acupuncture, on the other hand, utilizes thin needles to stimulate specific points in the body.

2. Method of Application

During an acupressure session, the practitioner applies gentle pressure to specific acupoints using their fingers, palms, or elbows. This technique resembles a soothing massage, where circular motions or pumping actions may be used. It's like a gardener pressing seeds into the soil, stimulating the energy to support plant growth.

In acupuncture, the practitioner carefully inserts thin needles into specific acupoints. This technique is comparable to a gardener skillfully pruning a plant, making precise cuts to encourage healthy growth. The needles are left in place for around 20 to 30 minutes, allowing you to relax while the process takes effect.

3. Conditions Treated

While acupressure and acupuncture can both be used to address a wide variety of health concerns, there are certain conditions where one might be preferred over the other. For instance, with its non-invasive approach, acupressure is often favored for stress relief, minor aches and pains, and overall wellness.

Acupuncture, on the other hand, is often used for more complex or chronic conditions, such as migraines, chronic pain, or infertility. However, the choice between acupressure and acupuncture largely depends on individual comfort levels, health needs, and preferences.

Remember, both techniques aim to harness and balance the body's Qi, fostering better health and wellness. They are different paths to the same destination - the serene garden of balanced energy and vibrant health.

Understanding Acupressure

Just as a skilled pianist precisely knows which keys to press to compose a beautiful melody, understanding acupressure points is vital in the symphony of acupressure therapy. These points, also known as "acupoints," are specific locations on the body along the meridians, or energy channels, where the Qi, or life energy, can be accessed and manipulated. These points have unique functions and therapeutic potential, like individual notes on a music sheet.

For example, the acupoint known as "He Gu" or "Large Intestine 4" is located on the hand, between the thumb and the index finger. It's often utilized to relieve headaches and pain. Applying gentle pressure to this point is like playing a specific note on the piano to bring harmony to the body's energetic composition. Acupressure is a simple yet effective way to tap into your body's natural healing abilities. With knowledge and practice, anyone can learn to use it for their well-being.

Self-Acupressure

Self-acupressure can be a personalized health toolkit you can take anywhere with you. This practice involves applying pressure to specific acupoints on your own body to help relieve discomfort or promote relaxation.

For instance, are you feeling a bit stressed out? Try massaging the "Ying Tang" point between your eyebrows, a technique often compared to hitting the 'refresh' button on your computer. Or, for a quick energy boost, you can stimulate the "Zusanli" point just below the knee.

Professional Acupressure Treatments

In contrast, when receiving professional acupressure treatment, you'll be guided through a carefully curated experience by a skilled practitioner who understands how to create a balanced and therapeutic session. In these sessions, a trained practitioner applies pressure to specific points on your body, often using their hands, fingers, or special instruments.

They might use various techniques, including pressing, kneading, tapping, or stretching your body. It's an opportunity to lie back and relax as the practitioner works to harmonize your energy flow.

Benefits and Risks

Acupressure offers many benefits that can bring comfort and relaxation. This practice is known to help reduce pain, decrease stress levels, improve sleep, enhance circulation, and even support digestive health. It's like having a toolbox filled with tools designed to handle different tasks easily and precisely.

While generally safe, individuals with specific health conditions such as heart disease, cancer, or pregnant women should consult with a healthcare professional before attempting acupressure. It's also worth noting that some people may experience temporary discomfort, light-headedness, or emotional release during or after an acupressure session.

Practical Application

Let's transform our understanding of acupressure into practical application, akin to a gardener finally sowing seeds after learning the gardening theory. Here are some simple acupressure techniques for common ailments:

- For headaches and migraines: Apply pressure to the "He Gu" (LI4) point between the thumb and index finger.

- For stress and anxiety: Massage the "Ying Tang" point between your eyebrows.

- For insomnia: Press the "Anmian" point on the back of the neck, just behind the ear.

- For indigestion: Stimulate the "Zusanli" (ST36) point, located about four finger-widths down from the bottom of your knee cap, along the outer boundary of your shin bone.

- For fatigue and low energy: Stimulate the "Zu San Li" (ST36) point, located on the lower leg, about four finger-widths below the kneecap, along the outer boundary of the shinbone.

- For back pain: Massage the "Huanzhong" point in the middle of the lower back between the two dimples above the buttocks.

Understanding Acupuncture

Acupuncture points are like pinpoints on a map of our bodies. They are distributed along energy pathways known as meridians, and each point has a specific purpose in maintaining our body's balance. For instance, "Shen Men" (HT 7) is a wrist point that might help with anxiety and insomnia. Another location on the lower leg, "Zu San Li" (ST36), can improve stamina and immunity.

An acupuncturist can alter the energy flow in your body by putting needles into certain spots, thereby restoring balance while encouraging well-being. They understand how to direct your body toward optimal health like an experienced guide navigates a journey.

Traditional Acupuncture

In this practice, the acupuncturist inserts thin, sterile needles into specific points on the body, following the guidelines set forth by ancient Chinese medicine. Much like a musician plucking a guitar string to produce a perfect note, the acupuncturist manipulates the needles to stimulate the body's Qi, encouraging the energy to flow harmoniously. It's a delicate symphony of precision and intuition, as each insertion plays a role in the broader healing melody of the body.

Electroacupuncture

Let's turn up the volume with electroacupuncture - it's like adding an electric guitar to a classic symphony. This modern adaptation of traditional acupuncture involves attaching a small, painless electrical device to the needles. The device delivers gentle electrical pulses, like rhythmic vibrations from a bass guitar, providing additional stimulation to the acupuncture points.

This method is often used when a stronger stimulation is desired, akin to amplifying a musical note for more impact in a song. Whether you choose the classical tones of traditional acupuncture or the amplified resonance of electroacupuncture, both techniques play in harmony to the tune of balanced Qi.

Benefits and Risks

Stepping into the realm of acupuncture brings a bouquet of potential benefits, like a welcoming breeze carrying the scent of blooming flowers. Studies have suggested that acupuncture may relieve various ailments, from chronic pain conditions such as arthritis and migraines to digestive disorders to mood-related issues like anxiety and depression.

While acupuncture is generally considered safe when performed by a trained practitioner, some people might experience mild side effects such as temporary soreness, light bleeding, or bruising at the needle sites.

Those with bleeding disorders, pacemakers, or pregnant women should discuss this with their healthcare provider before diving into acupuncture.

A bird's-eye view of potential benefits:

- Pain relief for conditions like arthritis, back pain, and migraines.

- Support for mental health, addressing issues like anxiety and depression.

- Relief from nausea and vomiting, particularly associated with chemotherapy.

- Improvement in sleep quality, potentially helping with insomnia.

Practical Application

Acupuncture can be applied to manage a variety of common ailments. However, as this practice involves the insertion of needles, it should always be performed by a trained professional. Before any acupuncture session, the practitioner will typically thoroughly evaluate your health status and personal needs. The treatment is then tailored to you, as unique as your fingerprint.

Here are some examples of how acupuncture can be utilized for various ailments:

- Chronic pain: The acupoints "He Gu" (LI4) and "Zu San Li" (ST36) are commonly stimulated to help relieve different types of pain, from headaches to joint pain.

- Stress and anxiety: The acupoint "Shen Men" (HT 7) is often targeted to alleviate stress and promote relaxation.

- Digestive issues: The acupoint "Zhong Wan" (RN 12) might be used to support digestive health.

- Insomnia: "An Mian" point, located near the ear, is a go-to for improving sleep.

Chapter Three
Aromatherapy and Essential Oils

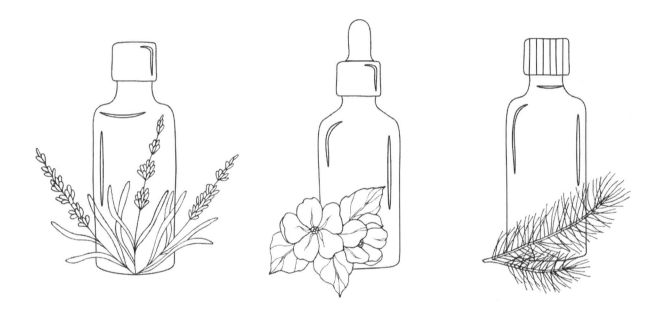

Aromatherapy, at its simplest, is a healing method that utilizes aromatic compounds derived from plants, commonly known as essential oils, to promote health and well-being. The term itself is relatively modern, coined by a French chemist named René-Maurice Gattefossé in the 1930s. However, using plant essences for therapeutic purposes traces its roots back thousands of years.

From the ancient Egyptians, who used aromatic plant materials in their spiritual rituals and cosmetics, to the Greeks and Romans, who employed them for medicinal and perfumery purposes, aromatherapy has a rich history intertwined with human civilization.

The principle behind aromatherapy is that the distinct aromas from these essential oils can stimulate our brain's limbic system - the area responsible for emotions and memory - thereby influencing our physical, emotional, and mental health. For instance, lavender oil is often used to induce a sense of calm and promote sleep, while citrus oils like lemon and orange are commonly used to energize and uplift.

In this therapeutic approach, something as simple as inhaling a particular aroma can act as medicine, gently guiding our bodies toward balance and wellness. As we venture further into aromatherapy, we will explore this fascinating interplay between scent, mind, and body in greater detail.

Understanding Essential Oils

Essential oils are the essence of a plant, the "soul," so to speak, captured in liquid form. Plants produce these oils for various reasons, such as to attract pollinators or repel pests, and they are typically stored in specific cells, ducts, or glandular hairs distributed among the plant's flowers, leaves, bark, stems, and roots. As these oils are incredibly concentrated, they encapsulate the fragrance and therapeutic properties of the plant from which they're derived.

Essential oils serve as the key ingredients in aromatherapy, enabling us to harness the healing power of plants in a concentrated and versatile form. For example, a single drop of rose essential oil is produced from about 30 roses, offering a rose garden's soothing and mood-lifting aroma in a single drop. Similarly, peppermint essential oil captures the invigorating scent of the peppermint plant, along with its cooling sensation and potential digestive benefits. However, because of their potency, they must be used with caution and respect for their powerful effects.

Extraction Methods

- Steam Distillation: This is the most common method of extracting essential oils. The plant material is placed into a still, and steam is passed through it. The heat causes the plant cells to break down and release their oils, evaporating into the steam. The steam and oil vapors are then condensed back into a liquid, separating the oil from the water.

- Cold Press Extraction: Mainly used for citrus oils like lemon, orange, or bergamot, the oil is squeezed out of the peel or rind under mechanical pressure. This method retains the vibrant, fresh scent of the fruit.

- Solvent Extraction: A solvent is used to extract the oils for plant materials that are too delicate for steam distillation, like jasmine or tuberose. The solvent dissolves the plant material, leaving a mixture of essential oil and waxy plant residues behind. This mixture, known as concrete, is further processed to remove the solvent, leaving behind what's known as an absolute.

- CO_2 Extraction: This very novel extraction process employs high-pressure carbon dioxide. When the pressure is decreased, the carbon dioxide evaporates, leaving the essential oil behind. This approach is ideal for conserving the delicate aroma compounds that heat can destroy in steam distillation.

- Enfleurage: This is an old and largely outdated method of extraction, traditionally used for delicate flowers like jasmine or lily. The flowers are spread on a fat-coated glass plate. The fat absorbs the oils from the flowers, and then alcohol is used to extract the oils from the fat.

Each of these extraction methods has its advantages and disadvantages, and the choice of method often depends on the type of plant and the properties of the oil to be extracted.

Categories of Common Essential Oils

In the diverse world of essential oils, you'll come across a plethora of categories, each with specific features and medicinal effects. While categorizing essential oils isn't an exact science, one popular way is to group them by their prominent notes or aroma categories - floral, citrus, woody, earthy, spicy, and herbaceous.

- Floral Oils: As the name suggests, these oils are distilled from flowers and carry a strong, sweet, and often romantic aroma. Lavender, an oil known for its calming effects, falls under this category. Similarly, Rose oil, with its rich, sensual scent, is hailed for its mood-boosting properties.

- Citrus Oils: These oils are typically cold-pressed from the rind of citrus fruits. They have bright, uplifting fragrances and are often used to alleviate feelings of anxiety and depression. Some common examples include Lemon, Orange, and Bergamot.

- Woody Oils: Extracted from trees or shrubs, these oils have a strong, grounding aroma, often used in meditation or for relaxation. With their warm, comforting scent, Cedarwood and Sandalwood, known for their deep, soft, woody fragrance, are popular choices in this category.

- Earthy Oils: Oils in this category possess a deep, heavy, soil-like scent. Vetiver and Patchouli are notable examples commonly used for grounding and creating a sense of calm.

- Spicy Oils: These oils have a warm, energizing aroma. They're often derived from seeds, bark, or roots of plants. Examples include Clove, which has a rich, spicy scent, and Cinnamon, appreciated for its sweet, warming aroma.

- Herbaceous Oils: These oils are reminiscent of green, leafy plants and herbs. They're typically fresh and crisp in scent. Peppermint, with its cooling, refreshing aroma, and Rosemary, with its strong, fresh, herbaceous scent, are part of this group.

Essential oils can be classified into several categories based on their complex aroma profiles. This variety adds to the depth of aromatherapy and makes it possible to make delightful combinations when oils are blended, resulting in an even broader range of therapeutic benefits.

How Aromatherapy Works

The essence of aromatherapy lies in its capacity to engage our senses, particularly our sense of smell, to trigger specific physiological responses and promote healing. Here, we will look at the mechanisms that underlie this intriguing process.

The Role of Smell in Healing

Unlike the rest of our senses, which are processed in the cerebral cortex, smell information travels directly to the limbic system, an area of the brain associated with emotions, memory, and certain physiological functions like heart rate and blood pressure. This direct pathway means scents can immediately impact our feelings and physical responses.

As the scent of a particular perfume may take you back to a memory of a person or place associated with that smell, similarly, the scent of lavender is frequently associated with relaxation and can induce feelings of calm almost instantly upon inhalation. This is the premise behind the use of essential oils in aromatherapy.

Moreover, research has shown that different scents can trigger different responses. Citrus scents like orange or lemon have been linked to increased alertness and improved mood. On the other hand, woody scents like cedarwood and sandalwood have been found to lower heart rate and blood pressure, indicating a relaxation response.

This deep connection between smell and our brain's emotional center allows aromatherapy to play a decisive role in healing. We can elicit certain emotional responses which help alleviate numerous mental and emotional health conditions, such as anxiety, depression, and insomnia, by carefully choosing and using essential oils.

In the same way, as the limbic system also controls certain physiological functions, the scents we inhale can directly impact our physical health. For instance, eucalyptus oil, when inhaled, is known to help clear congestion, making it a common choice during the cold and flu season.

The smell is a potent tool in the arsenal of natural healing, allowing us to manipulate our mood, improve our well-being, and even manage our physical health simply by choosing which scents to surround ourselves with. In this light, aromatherapy becomes an exploration of the sensory landscape, a journey into how our bodies respond to the fragrances of the natural world.

Methods of Application

Each application method offers its own benefits, and your choice can depend on your preferences, the type of ailment you wish to address, or even the specific essential oil you're using.

- Inhalation: The simplest and most direct method, inhalation, involves breathing in the oil's aroma, typically using a diffuser that disperses the oil into the air. Personal inhalers and steam inhalations are other popular ways to reap the benefits of essential oils through this method.

- Topical Application: Essential oils can be applied directly to the skin, but diluting them with a carrier oil is better and safer for preventing skin irritation. Common points of application include the wrists, temples, soles of the feet, or any specific area of concern.

- Bathing: A few drops of essential oil added to a warm bath creates an aromatic experience while also allowing the oils to be absorbed by the skin. It's an effective way to relax both the body and the mind after a long day.

- Massage: Massage allows for deeper penetration and absorption of the oils into the muscles and tissues. Before applying the essential oils, they are usually diluted with a carrier oil, which allows for a more effective and safer application.

- Internal Use: While some advocate for the internal use of essential oils, it's generally not recommended for beginners due to safety concerns. If choosing to ingest essential oils, it should always be under the guidance of a trained professional to ensure proper usage and dosage.

Commonly Used Essential Oils

Tea Tree: Originating from the leaves of the Melaleuca Alternifolia plant, tea tree oil is known for its potent antimicrobial properties. It's commonly applied topically to treat various skin conditions, including acne, fungal infections, and minor wounds. Additionally, it's used in aromatherapy for its purifying and cleansing effects and can support immune health.

- Chamomile: Well-known for its calming properties, chamomile oil is used to improve sleep, lower anxiety, and soothe skin irritations.

- Lavender: Derived from the lavender plant, this essential oil is renowned for its calming and soothing properties. It is often used to alleviate stress, promote relaxation, and enhance sleep. Lavender oil is also beneficial for skin health, frequently used to soothe skin irritations, minor burns, and insect bites.

- Lemon: Lemon essential oil is extracted from the peel of the citrus fruit and has a bright, refreshing aroma. It has been associated with improved mood, reduced stress, and enhanced memory. Its antibacterial qualities make it an outstanding natural cleaner, purifying surfaces and when used in a diffuser, even the air. Additionally, lemon oil has astringent properties that can help control oily skin and acne when used topically, so it can contribute to better skin.

- Peppermint: Peppermint oil is best known for its invigorating and refreshing effects. It's often utilized to calm headaches, reduce feelings of nausea, and promote clear breathing. Furthermore, it can relieve muscle aches due to its cooling effect.

- Rosemary: Derived from the popular culinary herb, rosemary essential oil carries a distinctive sharp, fresh, and herbaceous aroma. It stimulates mental activity, improves concentration, and supports respiratory health. Moreover, when diluted and applied topically, rosemary oil can help to alleviate muscle and joint pain, thanks to its anti-inflammatory and analgesic properties.

- Frankincense: Also known as the 'king of oils, frankincense has a warm, spicy aroma and is used to reduce feelings of stress and promote a sense of peace. It also supports skin health and has been used in meditative practices.

- Eucalyptus: With its crisp, clean aroma, eucalyptus oil is frequently used to support respiratory health. It can help clear nasal congestion, ease symptoms of a cough or cold, and has also been used to alleviate symptoms of allergies. In addition, its antibacterial properties make it a valuable oil for cleaning and purifying air.

- Bergamot: Bergamot oil has a distinctively fresh and uplifting aroma derived from a type of citrus fruit. It's frequently used in aromatherapy to alleviate stress, anxiety, and depression. Additionally, its antiseptic properties make it beneficial for skin conditions like acne.

- Ylang-Ylang: This essential oil, extracted from the flowers of the Cananga tree, has a sweet, floral aroma. Ylang-ylang oil is well-known for its mood-enhancing effects and is frequently used to treat stress, anxiety, and depression. It's additionally appreciated for its potential benefits to skin and hair health.

- Sandalwood: A timeless classic in aromatherapy, sandalwood oil is derived from the heartwood of the sandalwood tree. For its deep, serene, and woody aroma, it is often used to promote calm and relaxation, making it ideal for meditation. Furthermore, it's been used for skin care to help soothe and nourish the skin.

Making Aromatherapy Part of Your Daily Life

Incorporating aromatherapy into your daily life can be a joyful journey toward better health. This holistic practice can become an accessible, valuable part of your health and self-care routine with some essential tools and knowledge.

Aromatherapy Products

Numerous products are available that can help you integrate aromatherapy into your daily life. These, of course, are based on essential oils and can be utilized in their natural state, or they can be found in a variety of products like candles, lotions, bath salts, and even household cleaning products. Inhalers are a practical option for on-the-go use because they provide a quick, concentrated aroma. Scented body care products, like lotions or bath oils, offer an easy way to enjoy the benefits of essential oils while also nourishing your skin.

Then there are products designed to help diffuse the oils. Diffusers come in all shapes, sizes, and price ranges to disperse your chosen essential oil into the air for inhalation. Some use heat, while ultrasonic diffusers use water and sound waves. Each has its benefits, and your choice may depend on your specific needs and preferences.

DIY Essential Oil Recipes

If you enjoy a more hands-on approach, creating your aromatherapy products can be a fulfilling way to engage with essential oils. Making your own blends enables you to customize the aroma and therapeutic benefits to your needs and preferences. You can make a relaxing blend of lavender, chamomile, and frankincense for bedtime or a stimulating blend of peppermint and rosemary for when you need a boost of energy.

A wealth of resources is available, from books to online tutorials, to guide you in creating your own essential oil blends, candles, soaps, or body care products. Not only does this allow for customization, but it also ensures that you know what's in the products you're using.

Essential Oil Diffusers and Other Equipment

Essential oil diffusers work by dispersing essential oils into the air, creating a soothing aromatic environment. Several types of diffusers are available on the market, each with unique advantages.

- Nebulizing Diffusers: These diffusers work without heat or water. Instead, they use an atomizer to create fine particles of essential oils and release them into the air. They're often considered the most effective type of diffuser, providing a strong concentration of essential oils.

- Ultrasonic Diffusers: These diffusers use water and ultrasonic waves to diffuse essential oils. They double as humidifiers, making them an excellent choice for drier climates or use during the colder months when indoor air is dry.

- Heat Diffusers: These diffusers use heat from a candle or electricity to heat the oil and cause it to evaporate into the air. They are generally less expensive but less effective, as the heat can alter the chemical composition of the oils.

- Evaporative Diffusers: In these simple diffusers, a fan blows air through a pad or filter with essential oil, making the oil evaporate quickly. They are usually portable and simple to use. However, they may not release oils evenly in a large room.

Other tools, in addition to diffusers, could be helpful in your aromatherapy journey. Glass bottles for storing homemade blends, roller bottles for convenient oil application, and carrier oils for diluting are among them. Many accessories are available, including essential oil jewelry and portable inhalers, allowing you to indulge in the benefits of aromatherapy everywhere you go.

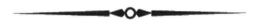

Exploring and experimenting with these options can turn aromatherapy into a daily ritual that enhances your quality of life, supporting your emotional and physical health. With a bit of practice and patience, these natural healing tools can offer a range of benefits, from stress relief and improved sleep to increased energy and physical well-being.

Chapter Four
Homeopathy

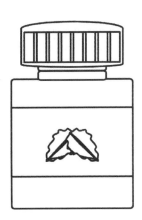 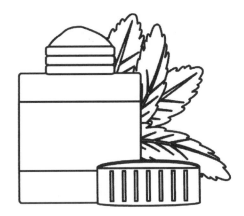 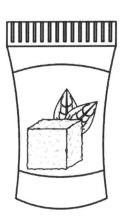

Homeopathy, a unique branch of natural medicine, holds an important place in the realm of healing, although it is often misunderstood. This form of alternative medicine, based on the principle of "like cures like," seeks to stimulate the body's innate healing mechanisms.

Derived from the Greek words "homoios," meaning similar, and "pathos," meaning suffering, homeopathy centers around the idea that substances causing symptoms in a healthy individual can, when diluted, treat similar symptoms in a sick person. It's an approach that emphasizes the holistic nature of health, addressing the individual as a whole rather than merely focusing on a specific disease's symptoms.

The origins of homeopathy can be traced back to the late 18th century, to the mind of a German physician named Samuel Hahnemann. He sought a more humane, effective healing method after becoming disappointed with the conventional medicine of the day, which often did more harm than good.

Homeopathy was born when Hahnemann while translating a medical treatise, questioned the then-accepted reason for why Cinchona bark (a malaria medication) was beneficial. He ingested the bark himself to examine and discovered that it caused symptoms comparable to malaria. The event set him on a path of investigation and discovery that resulted in the fundamental principles of homeopathy.

Key Principles of Homeopathy

The essence of homeopathy can be distilled into three primary principles. First, the Law of Similars, or "like cures like," is the bedrock of homeopathic philosophy. It suggests that a substance causing symptoms in a healthy person can cure similar symptoms in a sick person when administered in minute doses.

Second, the principle of the Minimum Dose highlights the practice of using the least amount of a substance needed to elicit a response. Homeopathic remedies are often diluted to such an extent that no molecules of the original substance remain. Yet, they are believed to retain a "memory" or "energy" that stimulates the body to heal itself.

Finally, the principle of the Single Remedy proposes that one remedy should cover all the physical, emotional, and mental symptoms the person is experiencing. This principle underscores the holistic view of homeopathy, emphasizing the interconnection of mind, body, and spirit.

Understanding the Homeopathic Approach

Understanding the enigmatic appeal of homeopathy begins with its central concept, Similia Similibus Curentur, or "like cures like." This concept reflects the belief that when taken in minute dosages, a substance that causes certain symptoms in a healthy person might alleviate identical or similar symptoms in a sick person.

The philosophy of "like cures like" turns our conventional understanding of disease and healing on its head. Where modern medicine frequently seeks to suppress symptoms, homeopathy interprets symptoms as the body's attempt to restore balance to heal itself. Thus, in the practice of homeopathy, symptoms are not enemies to be defeated and overcome but rather signposts directing us toward the appropriate remedy.

Imagine, for example, the common onion. Peeling an onion often brings tears to our eyes and may cause our noses to run. According to homeopathic principles, a remedy derived from the onion—Allium cepa—may treat conditions exhibiting similar symptoms, such as certain colds or allergies, where the person might experience watery eyes and a runny nose.

The Idea of the Minimum Dose

The concept of the minimum dose forms the second pillar of homeopathy. The essence of this idea lies in using the smallest possible amount of a medicinal substance to elicit healing. The practice embodies a respect for the body's inherent healing ability and reflects a desire to avoid side effects often associated with larger doses of medicinal substances.

But what is the 'minimum dose' in homeopathy? Homeopathic remedies undergo a unique serial dilution and succussion (vigorous shaking). A minute amount of the original substance—possibly a plant, mineral, or animal product—is diluted in water or alcohol and then succussed. This process is repeated multiple times, creating a highly diluted remedy. Some homeopathic medicines are so significantly diluted that they may not contain a single molecule of the original substance. Yet, homeopaths maintain that these remedies retain an energetic imprint of the initial material, sufficient to stimulate the body's healing response.

In homeopathy, a special process called potentization involves dilution and succussion. This process is believed to awaken the healing energy of the substance while minimizing side effects. Although controversial, the principle of the minimum dose adds to the intriguing nature of homeopathy.

The Concept of the Single Remedy

The final cornerstone of homeopathy is the principle of the single remedy. This idea is rooted in an individual's perception as a unified whole, where physical, mental, and emotional aspects are intimately interconnected.

In a homeopathic consultation, the practitioner observes the patient's physical complaints, feelings, disposition, personal habits, and even dreams. The remedy chosen is not targeted at a specific illness or a solitary symptom but at the entire individual, aiming to stimulate their inherent healing abilities.

For instance, let's consider two individuals suffering from migraines. In conventional medicine, both may be prescribed the same pain-relieving drug. However, in homeopathy, the treatment may differ for each. If one person experiences stress-related migraines, prefers cold environments, and feels better while resting, they may be prescribed one remedy. In contrast, if the other person has migraines triggered by hormonal changes, prefers warmth, and feels better while moving around, they may receive an entirely different remedy.

It is not the disease but how it manifests in the individual that guides the choice of the remedy in homeopathy. This personalized approach embodies the single remedy principle, which is integral to homeopathic philosophy and practice.

Prescribing a single remedy at a time allows the homeopaths to observe the effects of that particular remedy, ensuring it matches the totality of symptoms and individual characteristics of the patient. Thus, homeopathy upholds its commitment to understanding and treating each person as unique, reflecting the fundamental unity of mind, body, and spirit.

Homeopathic Remedies

The term "homeopathic remedies" may conjure images of quaint apothecary jars filled with exotic herbs. While this picture is partly accurate, it does not fully describe the depth and diversity of sources that make up homeopathic medicine. Homeopathic remedies tap into the innate power of nature, drawing upon a rich array of plants, minerals, and even animal products.

Plant-based remedies form a significant part of the homeopathic pharmacopeia. Some of these, like Allium cepa (red onion) or Arnica montana (mountain daisy), are familiar names, while others, like Stramonium (thorn apple) or Hyoscyamus (henbane), may sound more arcane.

Minerals, too, lend their unique properties to homeopathic remedies. Whether it's Ferrum phosphoricum derived from iron phosphate for a range of issues like inflammation or fatigue or Calcarea carbonica sourced from the middle layer of oyster shells often used for anxiety and digestive disorders, these remedies reflect the impressive breadth of the mineral kingdom.

Animal products also contribute to homeopathy's eclectic list of remedies. From the cuttlefish (Sepia) ink known to help balance hormonal issues, particularly in women, to the poison of the bushmaster snake (Lachesis) used for circulatory problems, these remedies underscore the remarkable range of homeopathy's sources.

Dilution and Potentization

Homeopathic medicines are more than just extracts from these organic sources. They go through a special dilution and potentization procedure that is utilized solely in homeopathy.

A typical process starts with a "mother tincture," a concentrated solution of the original substance in a mixture of water and alcohol. A drop might be taken from this tincture and added to 99 drops of a water-alcohol mixture. After vigorous shaking, the resulting diluted solution becomes a 1C potency. This method, known as succussion, is a common practice in homeopathy.

If one drop of the 1C potency is then taken and succussed with another 99 drops of the water-alcohol mixture, the result is a 2C potency. This serial dilution and succussion process can be continued, with potencies commonly seen in homeopathic practice ranging from 6C to 200C and beyond.

Following the principle of the minimum dose, remedies become energetically potent despite being materially diluted. The combination of dilution and succussion is believed to imprint the original substance's energetic pattern onto the water-alcohol mixture, making it therapeutically active while reducing adverse effects. The high-energy shaking that occurs during succussion differentiates homeopathy from other natural medicines.

Common Homeopathic Remedy Guide

Diving into the ocean of homeopathic remedies, we encounter a spectrum of healing possibilities. While each treatment is selected based on individual symptoms and constitution, certain remedies have been commonly used for specific ailments. These remedies are just a few examples out of thousands employed in homeopathy. Each remedy reflects a unique combination of symptoms and characteristics specific to an individual. Homeopaths match these remedies to a person's symptoms, aiming to support the body's natural healing processes and restore balance and well-being.

Here, we'll touch on a few notable examples to illustrate the breadth and scope of homeopathic medicine.

- Arnica Montana: Derived from a plant native to Europe, Arnica is one of the most recognized homeopathic remedies. Its powerful anti-inflammatory and analgesic properties have made it a go-to remedy for traumas, bruises, sprains, and muscle soreness.

- Nux Vomica: Extracted from the poison nut tree, Nux Vomica is often employed to treat digestive complaints. It's mainly associated with overindulgence in food or drink and may alleviate symptoms like heartburn, indigestion, or hangovers.

- Pulsatilla: Prepared from a plant called the windflower, Pulsatilla is frequently recommended for ailments with changing, inconsistent symptoms. It's commonly used in conditions relating to the ears, eyes, or the reproductive system, mainly where hormonal changes influence symptoms.

- Belladonna: Sourced from a highly toxic plant, the deadly nightshade, Belladonna, in its homeopathic form, is used for acute symptoms that come on suddenly. These could include high fever, throbbing headaches, or inflammation where the affected area appears red and feels hot.

- Apis Mellifica: This honeybee-derived medicine is frequently used for conditions characterized by swelling, redness, and stinging pain, similar to a bee sting. It can be used to treat skin issues, allergic reactions, and joint inflammation.

- Calcarea Carbonica: Made from the middle layer of oyster shells, Calcarea Carbonica is a remedy often suited to individuals with a slow metabolism who may feel overwhelmed and anxious. It's used for many symptoms, including fatigue, anxiety, and digestive or menstrual problems.

Application of Homeopathy

Homeopathy is fundamentally a holistic approach, viewing the individual as an interconnected whole rather than a collection of discrete components. As a result, homeopathy can address a wide range of acute and chronic health issues, encompassing the physical, emotional, and mental realms.

Physical ailments ranging from minor injuries, flu, allergies, and digestive disorders, to more chronic conditions such as arthritis, asthma, and skin conditions, are often addressed with homeopathy. Due to its gentle and non-toxic nature, it's also frequently used for children's ailments, including ear infections, teething troubles, and behavioral issues.

Homeopathy also addresses emotional and psychological issues. Homeopathic remedies have been utilized for treating anxiety, depression, stress-related problems, and even certain parts of autistic spectrum disorders. The appealing characteristic of homeopathy is its capacity to adapt treatment to each individual's symptom profile and constitutional type.

However, while homeopathy can significantly manage a vast range of health conditions, it doesn't mean that it can entirely replace the need for conventional medical diagnosis or treatment, particularly in severe chronic diseases. It can, nevertheless, work in conjunction with traditional therapies to support overall well-being.

Procedure for a Homeopathic Consultation

A homeopathic consultation is a one-of-a-kind experience distinguished by its depth and adaptation. Rather than focusing exclusively on the disease, the homeopath examines the individual's condition experience, getting a deep understanding of their symptoms and their impact on the individual's life.

During the consultation, the homeopath will ask different questions, which can include detailed descriptions of physical symptoms, personal and family medical history, lifestyle habits, food preferences, sleep patterns, and emotional state. The goal is to comprehensively understand the individual's health and life situation. This picture serves as a roadmap for selecting the most suitable homeopathic remedy.

Choosing the best treatment is a difficult task. The homeopath will analyze the information gathered during the consultation and will match the individual's symptom profile to a remedy's "proving" profile (the range of symptoms a remedy is known to have generated in healthy patients during clinical trials). The remedy that best matches the totality of the person's symptoms is finally decided.

Success Stories and Criticisms of Homeopathy

Navigating through the annals of homeopathy, we encounter numerous anecdotes of healing, where individuals report significant improvements in their health and well-being following homeopathic treatment. Success stories range from rapid recovery from acute conditions like flu and minor injuries to substantial improvements in chronic diseases like eczema, arthritis, or anxiety disorders. Some parents testify to the beneficial effects of homeopathy in addressing their children's health issues, from teething troubles to childhood eczema or behavioral difficulties.

However, homeopathy encounters its fair share of criticism alongside these success stories. Skeptics argue that homeopathy lacks robust scientific evidence supporting its efficacy, pointing to studies that show no significant difference between homeopathic remedies and placebos. The concept of ultra-high dilutions, a fundamental principle of homeopathy, has also drawn scrutiny. Critics question how a remedy diluted beyond Avogadro's number (where potentially not a single molecule of the original substance remains) could still possess therapeutic effects.

In response, homeopaths and researchers in the field refer to a growing body of research, including laboratory studies, animal studies, and clinical trials, suggesting that homeopathic remedies have effects beyond placebo. They also point to theories from the field of quantum physics, which suggest that water may have the ability to retain information from substances with which it has been in contact, providing a possible explanation for the action of highly diluted remedies.

It's worth noting that, despite ongoing debates, homeopathy enjoys widespread use all over the world, with millions of people relying on it for their healthcare needs. Many people who use homeopathy admire its holistic approach, customized treatment, and lack of side effects that are common with conventional medications.

While homeopathy continues to spark curiosity and controversy, we cannot deny its enduring appeal and its potential to play a complementary role in our healthcare landscape. Its individualistic approach, respect for the body's innate healing capacity, and the breadth of its remedy sources make homeopathy a fascinating chapter in the broad book of natural medicine.

Homeopathy and the Holistic Healing Practices

With its holistic approach and respect for the body's innate healing capacities, homeopathy fits seamlessly into the broader landscape of holistic healing practices. It often works hand-in-hand with various other modalities to facilitate an individual's journey to wellness.

In holistic health, nutrition plays a significant part, working together with homeopathic treatment. For instance, individuals with chronic digestive complaints may receive a homeopathic remedy that matches their specific symptoms and guidance on adjusting their diet.

Likewise, mind-body practices like yoga and meditation can enhance the effects of homeopathic treatment. For instance, a person suffering from anxiety may benefit from a homeopathic remedy by incorporating regular mindfulness meditation into their routine.

Integrating homeopathy with other holistic practices reinforces the concept of integrative health, which is a multidisciplinary approach that aims to use the most effective solutions for each individual's health needs. This collaborative approach facilitates a more complete and personalized pathway to wellness.

Current Trends in Homeopathy

Current trends in homeopathy reflect its growing acceptance and integration into mainstream healthcare. Homeopathic remedies for self-care for minor, self-limiting conditions are on the rise. Remedies for common ailments like colds, flu, minor injuries, and simple digestive complaints can be found in health food stores and some pharmacies, allowing individuals to proactively manage their health.

On a larger scale, there are increased efforts to conduct robust scientific research in homeopathy to provide solid evidence for its efficacy. Observational studies, clinical trials, and research exploring possible mechanisms of action for homeopathic remedies are part of an ongoing endeavor to build a substantial body of scientific literature on homeopathy.

Homeopathy is also gaining popularity among conventional healthcare practitioners. Homeopathy courses are accessible for doctors, nurses, and pharmacists who want to broaden their treatment options. The growing acceptance of homeopathy by the professional healthcare community suggests a shift toward a more holistic approach to healthcare.

The Future of Homeopathy

Looking ahead, the future of homeopathy seems promising. With an increasing number of people seeking natural, personalized healthcare options, homeopathy has the potential to become an even more significant player in the health and wellness field.

Integrating homeopathy into conventional healthcare systems is a potential avenue for the future. This would involve collaboration between homeopaths and traditional healthcare providers to provide the best possible care for each individual. Technological advancements may also influence the future of homeopathy. From online consultations to apps that help individuals select self-care remedies, technology is expanding the reach of homeopathy.

Ongoing research is vital in advancing our understanding of homeopathy and its potential applications in healthcare. Through rigorous scientific investigation, researchers aim to unravel the mechanisms underlying the therapeutic effects of homeopathic remedies, further explore their principles, and identify the specific conditions or patient populations that may benefit the most. This ongoing scientific investigation serves to develop and improve homeopathic practice, ensuring its relevance and effectiveness in addressing a wide range of health conditions. By continuously expanding our knowledge through research, we can reach the full potential of homeopathy and its contribution to holistic healthcare.

CONCLUSION

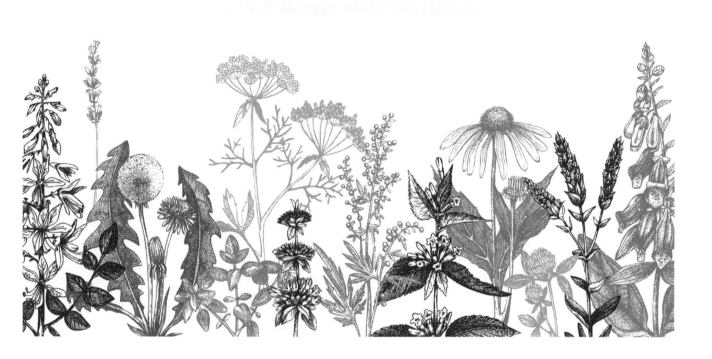

As we come to the end of this book, let's take a moment to reflect on the profound impact of herbal remedies in our lives. From the simple act of sipping herbal tea to the captivating aromas of essential oils, these remedies connect us to the power of nature's healing potential. However, our exploration into the world of herbal remedies doesn't stop here. The journey continues, and there is always more to learn and discover. Embrace the path of lifelong learning, whether through courses, books, or engaging with fellow herbal enthusiasts. Let your curiosity lead you deeper into the fascinating realm of herbal wisdom.

As you deepen your understanding, pay attention to the subtle connections between nature, herbs, and your own body. These connections are key to unlocking profound insights and guiding you toward holistic well-being. Holistic health is about recognizing the intricate interplay between our physical, mental, and emotional well-being. It's like a symphony, where each aspect harmonizes to create a beautiful and balanced melody. Every element contributes to the symphony of well-being, from herbal remedies to nourishing food, from mindfulness practices to physical movement. Embrace this holistic approach to health and allow it to infuse every aspect of your life. Trust in the innate wisdom of nature and the healing potential within yourself.

Let me tell you that your health journey is a vibrant dance celebrating the gift of life. As we close this chapter, know that the book may end, but your journey toward optimal health and wellness continues. With each step, you grow, evolve, and become more attuned to the wisdom of herbs and your own body's needs. The realm of herbal remedies is vast and full of possibilities. Embrace the adventure, explore with curiosity, and let the beauty of holistic health unfold in your life. Here's to a future filled with vibrancy, balance, and well-being.

I also want to take a moment to express my heartfelt gratitude to you. Thank you for embarking on this journey of herbal remedies and holistic health with me. Your dedication to expanding your knowledge and embracing natural healing approaches is genuinely inspiring. By exploring the pages of this book, you have shown a commitment to nurturing your well-being and connecting with the power of nature's remedies.

I hope that the information shared within these chapters has provided valuable insights and practical guidance, sparking a sense of curiosity within you. May this newfound knowledge empower you to make informed choices for your health and well-being and guide you on a path of vibrant, healthy living. Here's to a life filled with vitality, balance, and wellness!

Thanks

T hank you for reading "The Herbal Remedies Bible". By choosing to explore the wonders of natural medicine, you've taken a step towards holistic wellness.

Special Gift Just For You! To express our deepest gratitude, we are thrilled to offer an exclusive FREE BONUS: **"The Herbal A-Z"** - An Indispensable Guide to Over 200 Medicinal Plants. Uncover more healing secrets by scanning the QR code below.

We sincerely hope "The Herbal Remedies Bible" has enriched your understanding for natural remedies. If this guide has inspired you, we'd be truly honored if you could share your thoughts with a review on Amazon. Every piece of feedback not only illuminates the path for potential readers but also fuels our dedication to producing even more enlightening content for you.

Once more, thank you for being a part of our passionate community. Your support means the world to us!

References

In this section, I have compiled a list of valuable sources that have enriched our understanding of the topics covered in this book.

- Green, J. (2000). The Herbal Medicine-Maker's Handbook: A Home Manual. Crossing Press.

- Hoffmann, D. (2003). Medical Herbalism: The Science and Practice of Herbal Medicine. Healing Arts Press.

- McIntyre, A. (2010). The Complete Herbal Tutor: The Ideal Companion for Study and Practice. Gaia.

- Gladstar, R. (2012). Rosemary Gladstar's Medicinal Herbs, Storey Books

- Mills, S., & Bone, K. (2013). Principles and Practice of Phytotherapy: Modern Herbal Medicine. Churchill Livingstone.

- Horne, S. & Easley, T. (2016). The Modern Herbal Dispensatory, North Atlantic Books

- Chevallier, A. (2016). Encyclopedia of Herbal Medicine. DK Publishing.

- Cech, R. (2016). Making Plant Medicine, Herbal Reads LLC

- De La Foret, R. (2017). Alchemy of Herbs: Transform Everyday Ingredients into Foods & Remedies That Heal, Hay House Inc.

- Davis, C. & Apelian N. (2019). The Lost Book of Herbal Remedies, Global Brother

- De la Foret, R. & Han, E. (2020). Wild Remedies: How to Forage Healing Foods and Craft Your Own Herbal Medicine, Hay House Inc.

- Blankespoor, J. (2022). The Healing Garden: Cultivating and Handcrafting Herbal Remedies, Harvest

Made in the USA
Las Vegas, NV
25 October 2023

79564402R00120